Praise for Change Your Mind, Change Your Health

"Annie has proven herself in the industry as someone to listen to when making personal lifestyle changes. This is a must read for those interested in making and sustaining their own health & well-being changes, and in helping others throughout the behavior change process."

—Dee W. Edington, PhD, Professor Emeritus University of Michigan, author of Zero Trends coauthor of Health as a Win-Win Organizational Philosophy

D0011453

CHANGE YOUR MIND, CHANGE YOUR HEALTH

7 WAYS TO HARNESS THE POWER OF YOUR BRAIN TO ACHIEVE TRUE WELL-BEING

BY ANNE MARIE LUDOVICI, MS

New Page Books
A Division of The Career Press, Inc.
Pompton Plains, NJ

CHANGE YOUR MIND, CHANGE YOUR HEALTH
EDITED AND TYPESET BY GINA SCHENCK
Cover design by Joanna Williams Design
Printed in the U.S.A.

To order this title, please call toll-free 1-800-CAREER-1 (NJ and Canada: 201-848-0310) to order using VISA or MasterCard, or for further information on books from Career Press.

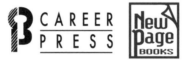

The Career Press, Inc.
220 West Parkway, Unit 12
Pompton Plains, NJ 07444
www.careerpress.com
www.newpagebooks.com

Library of Congress Cataloging-in-Publication Data
Ludovici-Connolly, Anne Marie, 1959-
  Change your mind, change your health : 7 ways to harness the power of your brain to achieve true well-being / by Anne Marie Ludovici, MS ; foreword by Dr. James O. Prochaska.
    pages cm
  Includes bibliographical references and index.
  ISBN 978-1-60163-344-6 (paperback) -- ISBN 978-1-60163-438-2 (ebook)
1. Self-care, Health. 2. Well-being. 3. Mind and body. 4. Health--Psycholog-ical aspects. I. Title.

RA776.95.L84 2014
613--dc23
                                                                    2014036118

This book is dedicated to my son, Kyle Mark Connolly, who has, and continues to, transform me and my life in the most amazing way! Kyle, you are, and always will be, my "Sunshine."

Acknowledgments

I am deeply grateful for all of the members, clients, groups, organizations, employers, colleagues, and friends that I have had the pleasure of working with throughout my 30-year career in the health and wellness industry. Each one of you has made significant contributions to my experiences, career, this book, and my personal well-being. Thank you to the brilliant researchers who have devoted their careers and lives to the continued work in the development and application of the behavior change theories, strategies, techniques, and tools presented in this book. You have improved the health and well-being of populations across the globe.

I especially want to thank Dr. James O. Prochaska, for his important work on the Transtheoretical Model of behavior change. Dr. Prochaska, I am grateful and humbled by your mentorship, collaboration, and councel throughout the years, for writing the Foreword, and for providing such an insightful and pertinent review of this book. Thank you to Dr. Janice Prochaska for her valuable insights and edits. And my sincere gratitude and appreciation to Jan and Jim for their continued support and friendship.

I am very appreciative to my "Super Agent," Jeff Herman, for believing in this book, and in me, and for taking me on as a client. You have literally helped me make a dream come true. I also want to thank Deb Herman for her critical edits to the book proposal and getting me started on social media. Thank you to Career Press/New Page Books for publishing this book and for your support.

Special acknowledgments go to Dr. Kathleen Cullinen, my doctoral and senior editor, content advisor in population-based health promotion, and dear friend. I can't thank you enough for your support though a *second* book! You have helped make the content shine as bright as the shining star you are! Thank you to Eva-Molly Pettito-Dunbar, doctoral student in psychology at University of Rhode Island, for providing the most up-to-date research citations, and for conceptual support. I am grateful to Donna Ingram, my longtime friend and research associate, for your content contributions. Thanks to Tim Marran for his creative additions, as well as editing support to the book proposal. And, to Charles, from Charles Desper Designs, thank you for all your creative design work for my Website and illustrations for this book. And, thanks to Big River Advertising for their awesome catalog copy, author's bio, and blog content used in this publication.

Last but not least, I am ever indebted to my family. Sincere thanks to my husband, Greg, my trusted advisor, and biggest "cheerleader." Your wisdom, support, and patience throughout this journey and our life journey together is so precious to me. A big thanks to my talented son, Kyle, for his love and encouragement throughout my career and this process. Kyle, I am so proud of you! And to my late first husband, Mark J. Connolly, the father of our son, Kyle, the greatest gift of all. Mark, you are missed. Special acknowledgments go to my beloved, late father, who motivates me daily with his never-to-be forgotten traits of perseverance, self-discipline and true Grit. Thank you to my mom, who always encouraged me to follow my dreams, and provided me with the "verbal persuasion" to achieve them. You gave it your all, exemplified true grit, and as a result, your cancer is in complete remission! Mom, I am so proud of you! Heartfelt acknowledgments go to my late brother, Dino, my memories of whom remind me to be more like the kind, compassionate, and gentle soul that he was. Thank you to my uncle, Ed Pereira, artist extraordinaire, for your help with countless versions of book cover designs for past book proposals. Thank you to my late grandparents, my "second" parents. My grandmother (*Avóa*) imparted such grace, wisdom, and love that warm my soul to this day. And finally, I express my gratitude for the lifelong, personal impact of my grandfather (*Avô*), my role model and a trailblazer of health, well-being, and personal achievement!

With Gratitude and Love, Anne Marie (Annie) Ludovici-Connolly

Contents

Foreword

Only Anne Marie Ludovici could have written this book. Only Annie could have presented the principles of high impact programs from so many intriguing perspectives. She writes from painful experiences of a health club owner who watched too many start a program only to stop too soon. From Club Med in the Caribbean she reports her overly cautious concerns that exercising in the sand could cause accidents. While she tried to gather a few Club Med members into her indoor encounters, she watched as a large crowd danced down the beach modeling their Caribbean coach. Lesson learned—wellness can be fun, and in this book Annie makes it fun.

Annie writes as a national consultant for a major health benefits company. She is often surprised at how some major employers are poorly informed of the importance of evidence-based programs. They often have only average wellness programs, despite evidence available that demonstrates how average programs perform poorly. Then they conclude that wellness programs don't work—at least not very well. But, based on the best practices, wellness programs can work very well. So, Annie presents the best practice principles that can help you change your mind so you can change your health.

Annie writes with such enthusiasm, such humor, such warmth and wisdom with insightful and inspiring stories that are worth the price of admission. The wellness field has learned all too loudly that engaging individuals in average programs is a huge challenge. More and more employers have turned to paying their employees growing amounts of money for participating in programs. Or, they are penalizing employees even greater amounts if they don't participate.

No one is paying you to buy and apply the principles in this book. So Annie's first principle of engagement is that this book needs to be fun. If Annie reminds you of Richard Simmons, you won't be the first one. Annie is not a celebrity—at least not yet. But, she does bring glamour to her repertoire. Besides dancing at Club Med, she shares stories of a rock star singing on a cruise who is faced with anxieties over not performing effectively enough. From Newport, Rhode Island, she seeks to help a top competitor in the famous America's Cup sailing races to loosen up on the town. But, she ends up admiring his discipline and his commitment to being the best prepared he can be.

Annie displays plenty of style along with some of the fads and fashions that come and go in wellness. But there is also plenty of substance supported by facts as Annie presents a striking line-up of best practice principles. She starts with our Transtheoretical Model, which is designed to provide an integrative framework for constructs from across leading theories of behavior and behavior change—hence the name Transtheoretical. She starts with our stages of change and helps you to appreciate how change principles from different theories can be best applied at particular stages of change.

With special expertise in Al Bandura's self-efficacy theory, Annie makes easily accessible the behavioral keys to mastery that build your confidence so that you can keep progressing in the face of very challenging and tempting situations. She then turns to cognitive keys that can unlock beliefs that are deeply embedded in your brain. You can open your mind to ways of thinking that can guide you to where you want to be and remove ways of thinking that get in your way.

Annie then draws on her experience in successfully managing a business and applies best business practices to help you better manage your life. Making a new life plan reflects the lesson learned that wellness at its best isn't just changing behaviors. It's really changing lives. She also provides a personal perspective of lessons learned from her grandfather from Portugal on how to best manage her weight.

From Newport, Annie returns to her challenges of coaching high-performance athletes in the highly competitive America's Cup races. Being able to be tough-minded is essential to get through tough times. The saying was that if the United States lost the America's Cup to another country, the Cup on the pedestal in the New York Yacht Club would have to be replaced by the head of the losing Captain. From the perspective of sports psychology, Annie makes it clear that successful behavior change is more mental than physical. As a coach and as an author, she provides a sensitive balance between being tough-minded and tender-hearted. She also is a wonderful model for staying positive even in the face of failure, loss, or setbacks.

Annie again shares her personal loss of her husband as an example of how major life events can challenge our commitment to living well. Such events can shake our self-efficacy and challenge our mental toughness. They can lead to lapses but do not have to produce relapses, if we have internalized the lessons learned from the time spent being tutored by Annie.

When life threatens to push us to our limits, we will be prepared to push back if we have internalized Annie's last lesson. If we have made the efforts to develop our grit, our perseverance, and passion for a goal like living well, then we will have the grit and resilience to endure times of suffering and struggling without letting go of our goal to live a life that is thriving.

This Foreword reflects the fact that there are huge differences in the success rates across wellness programs and among wellness professionals. There also are major differences in the impacts of self-help books and the authors who produce such books. I have given equal emphasis to the high-impact principles applied in this book and to the special author who functions like a master coach, teacher, consultant, counselor, and friend. In your journey to change your mind and enhance your health you are in the hands of one of my favorite friends and colleagues in the wellness field.

—James O. Prochaska, PhD, author, *Changing for Good*,
director of the Cancer Prevention Research Center, University of
Rhode Island, and founder and consultant to Pro-Change Behavior
Systems, Inc.

Introduction

IT'S TIME
It's time to change.
Time to turn over a new leaf,
To transform your health and well-being,
To live your life with vitality, meaning and energy,
To be YOU, but even BETTER and...to THRIVE.
It's time to *Change Your Mind, Change Your Health!*

If you picked up this book, you may know it's time, but you may be wondering, if *this time* you be successful at changing your health and sustaining the change you are striving for, yearning for, and desiring to improve your health and well-being. The time to improve your health is now, and this book can help you succeed *this time*!

> *"Time and health are two precious assets that we don't recognize and appreciate until they have been depleted."*
> —Denis Waitley

It's no secret: Change is difficult. Everyone knows it. Yet we all often wish to change something about our personal health behaviors, habits, or lifestyles. Fortunately, the real secret is that meaningful, successful, and sustainable change *is* possible, once you know how.

Change is a process of transformative self-enrichment that is easier once you know how to successfully undertake the change you wish to achieve. The problem is most people simply don't have the right tools, resources, or knowledge of how health behavior change works *for them*. After all, behavior change is a very personal experience. Celebrity diets and cookie-cutter fads don't work for everyone, but we often assume they do. And when they don't work for you, you think you've failed and you give up. But you haven't failed; you simply didn't discover the right approach for you, and/or used the proper techniques to set yourself up for success!

A Flight of Theories

The evidence-based health behavior change theories, self-assessments, strategies, techniques, tools, and tips presented in *Change Your Mind, Change Your Health* represent a "flight" of the world's finest health behavior change theories applied today worldwide! As a flight of wine allows tasting of multiple varieties, as well as an opportunity learn a bit about the wines, *Change Your Mind, Change Your Health* will provide a sampling of the best proven or evidence-based behavior change theories. Although there are other evidence-based theories of behavior change in related disciplines, such as health psychology and neuropsychology, the "sampling" selected specifically for this book will help you get started and help you continue to be successful on your personal journey of change.

Research has shown that only about 20 percent of the population is preparing to change or take action at any given point of time. Rest assured you are not alone if you are *not* ready for action at the beginning of your journey. *Change Your Mind, Change Your Health* will help you change in *your* way and at *your* pace to transform your health and your life. Its goal is for you to achieve an independent, self-assured, and sustainable sense of health and well-being in the face of all obstacles or challenges. Sometimes, we jump into action without taking time to prepare for unpredictable or "lifecycle" events that we will encounter at some point in our lives. In fact, research has shown that only 20 percent of the population actually conquers a long-term problem behavior and reaches maintenance of their new, positive behavior on the first attempt.

Without the appropriate "prep time" and leveraging the right strategies at the right time, we are setting ourselves up for a greater likelihood of failure.

Change Your Mind, Change Your Health will reveal "7 Ways to Harness the Power of Your Brain to Achieve True Well-Being" through theories, self-assessments, strategies, techniques, tools, and tips used by health behavior change experts, researchers, health coaches, and other health and psychology professionals. These seven ways, or "Insider Secrets," that behavior change experts use to move people toward permanent change will become clear and evident to you as you put them into practice. The strategies and techniques will provide you with a comprehensive toolbox that can be tailored to serve as a personal coach as you learn how to intrinsically motivate yourself to move toward and sustain behavior change to reach your health goals. You will identify your personal barriers to successful behavior change in your life as you implement strategies to minimize or permanently remove them. Through detailing the "Insider Secret" approaches used in the field of health behavior change, this book is designed to inspire you to move toward positive health behaviors and permanent change. Oh, and I almost forgot the most important part: You'll have fun in the process!

As a national health and well-being consultant and designer of health programs for major corporations and organizations, I bring firsthand evidence that the biggest problem for well-intentioned participants is not the wellness programs offered, but the inability to engage and *adhere* to the proper programs that allow for permanent and sustainable changes.

"Do you know what you should do to change your poor health habits?" I asked the participants in the behavior change study on weight loss that I conducted for my master's thesis. A stunning 98 percent of the group said, "Yes." They replied they knew what they should do to change, but confessed they just don't do it.

Colleen, a participant in my behavior change study, is a great example. Being a nurse, she knew exactly what healthy eating and physical activity behaviors consisted of. She would start a program, stick to it for a while, lose weight, then—for various reasons—slide back into her former eating habits and sedentary lifestyle. She experienced this pattern so many times that she believed she would never succeed in permanently changing her poor lifestyle behaviors.

Unfortunately, statistics support her belief; one third of Americans who eat healthy and are physically active for a period of time gain back all the weight they lost and sometimes more. Information on nutrition and physical activity is more plentiful than ever before. People are also more educated about health and fitness than ever before, yet obesity is at an all-time high with new reports claiming that more than 80 percent of our U.S. adult population is overweight or obese. The diet industry is a 60-billion-dollar industry. If people are spending more money each year, they are cleary aware and educated about improving their health and wellness then ever before. Then why are these health statistics demonstrating that all the current books and plans aren't working?

It is clear that poor health due to lifestyle behaviors is a global issue as well. The World Health Organization revealed that eight modifiable health risks and behaviors drive 15 chronic conditions that account for 80 percent of total costs of all chronic illnesses worldwide. Most of these costs and conditions are controllable by changing lifestyle habits. Usually, it's not the nutrition, physical activity, smoking cessation, or stress managment program that's flawed; the mistake is the individual's attempt to change poor lifestyle habits *without* sufficient knowledge of effective strategies and techniques for permanent change! More importantly, many don't know how to change, what change really means, and how to sustain change over time. Behavior change is not an event of changing a lifetime of poor health behaviors that one simply wakes up to one day. This "quick fix" way of thinking is the main cause of relapse or not sustaining behavior change. Research and behavior change experts have discovered that change is really a process, a personal journey, and not a destination or an event. Once one can truly embrace what change means and how to embark on a personal journey, he or she can form realistic self-expectations, be less demoralized, and more empowered!

Some of the Insider Secrets, or components of them, may seem familiar. However, knowing the theory behind them and understanding the full rationale can help you lead an empowered life, restructured with the same tools effective practitioners use. You will learn the rationale behind the processes and techniques as well as having practical self-assessments and activities to put these proven scientific behavior change theories into successful practice. If you are contemplating change and are ready to change your life once and for all for the better, this is a place to start. This is not another diet book that tells you *what* you need to do, without revealing *how* to go about it. When it is a lifetime of poor health habits that someone is trying to change, the "how" is the most important part of the process. This book is a blueprint that is partially designed for you. It is not a one-size-fits-all, because your health behaviors, needs, supports, barriers, and situations are not the same as anyone else's. The self-management and self-leadership approach to health behavior change enable you to take charge of how you start, proceed, and sustain your lifelong personal journey.

I have spent the last 30 years of my career applying evidence-based theories of change to myself and others. I share these applications with you because I know that anyone who is committed to achieving lifelong health and well-being *can* achieve it. The approaches shared in *Change Your Mind, Change Your Health* lead to invigoration, empowerment, and meaningful living through *intrinsic* motivation and increased confidence or self-efficacy. I share my personal life experiences, including the challenges and struggles I have faced, and continue to face, while maintaining positive health behaviors. It was, in fact, my own personal challenges that fueled my passion to study behavior change and cultivated the drive to inspire others to reap the innumerable benefits of change as well. My stories are gleaned from my personal life and professional work in health behavior change as a national consultant and expert in the health and wellness field. This includes my work at Club Med Resorts, training the America's Cup Crews, all the way to the inner workings of corporate America.

Change Your Mind, Change Your Health will guide you step-by-step to conquer your challenges and reveal your power to change your life for good. Like Dorothy in *The Wizard of Oz*, she discovered the power of her ruby slippers, realizing she had the power within her all along....

Journal Your Journey

Throughout this book, there are Journal Activities, as well as Action Items at the end of each chapter. I suggest you use this book as a workbook of sorts, to document your journey of change. Journaling or personal diary work has been shown to enhance progress and outcomes related to the successful achievement of goals for behavior change. You can use a regular notebook or purchase a "special" journal, or one with motivational quotes for further inspiration. Journaling helps you reflect on your thoughts, actions, and progress. It allows you to look back to remind you of successes, and how you pushed through change during the most difficult times of your life. Journaling may assist you in identifying your thought and lifestyle patterns while working through barriers to change. By giving your complete focus, thought, and refection of progress and challenges, it is a widely accepted and recommended technique for self-motivation and self-monitoring of successful long-term health behavior change.

It works if you work it."
—slogan from Alcoholics Anonymous

I would like to encourage you to work this program so it works for you by actively performing and completing all of the journal activities, assessments, and action items presented. This program, like any other, will only work if *you* work it.

Let your change begin!

Part I

Making the Change:
7 Insider Secrets for Permanent Change

1

Am I Ready to Change?

Insider Secret #1:
The "Stages of Change"

There is more to changing than just waking up and saying, "Today is the day!" It is a meaningful process of transformative self-enrichment. Imagine a room filled with unlit candles. You light one and things begin to become apparent. You start seeing things you never noticed before. You might become more aware of, or in touch with, feelings inside of you. As you light more and more candles, you become bathed in a new, warm glow. You have not only illuminated yourself, you have illuminated your world.

We will begin your illuminating journey of change by introducing you to the "Stages of Change." Stages of Change are part of the Transtheoretical Model of Behavior change (TTM) developed by Dr. James O. Prochaska and Dr. Carlo C. DiClemente, both internationally recognized researchers in the field of health behavior change. Their work is being used by researchers and practitioners worldwide, and in a variety of settings, to help people understand how they change and to provide them with evidence-based strategies to assist their clients with achieving and maintaining positive health behaviors. (Strategies or interventions that have the potential to affect individual behavior have been substantiated by evaluation, the results of which have been published in a peer-reviewed journals.)

The Transtheoretical Model encompasses several behavior change theories, thus the name transtheoretical (or integrating across theories).

When I first heard the term *Transtheoretical Model*, it sounded very intimidating to me. However, once I learned more about it, I found it to be very applicable to my life and to the lives of my clients. In fact, the model is easy to understand, is easy to apply, and has demonstrated amazingly positive and effective changes across multiple behaviors. The model includes four main constructs or components: Stages of Change, Processes of Change, Decisional Balance, and Self-Efficacy. All four of these components will be discussed and applied throughout this book.

Although it is important to embrace one's desire to change, one of the first steps is to know just what Stage of Change one is in. Because Stage of Change is the best predictor of a person's readiness to change, it is the best place to begin your journey. This chapter will guide you through understanding the six Stages of Change: *precontemplation, contemplation, preparation, action, maintenance,* and *termination*. It also includes a self-assessment to help you determine which Stage of Change you are currently in for the health behavior that you would like to change or improve. "Stage of Change predicts the likelihood of success in people's change attempts more accurately than anything else about them" (Prochaska, Norcross, and DiClemente, 2002).

As a personal and organizational consultant in the field of health behavior change, I have trained health coaches on the application of behavior change theories and techniques for their health and clinical practices, including how to apply the Stages of Change. Lisa, a health coach I worked with, asked me for advice on a particular client who was having difficulty maintaining the plan she put in place to help. Joe, her client, told Lisa he wanted to improve his eating habits and was ready to change, yet he was not following her recommendations. When I asked Lisa what Stage of Change her client was in, she told me he was in the *action* stage and ready for change.

Because Joe told Lisa he was ready to change, it was reasonable to assume he was in the *action* stage. However, after I asked Lisa to complete a Stage of Change assessment with Joe, Lisa discovered Joe was actually in the *contemplation* stage, requiring a very different coaching approach. Although Joe stated he wanted to improve his eating habits, he was not ready to act on his desire to change. That explained why Joe wasn't achieving his coach's anticipated results. Knowing her client's correct stage, *contemplation*, Lisa could now tailor Joe's plan to guide him appropriately along the stage continuum to achieve progress and/or improvements in his eating habits.

"Change means progress, not necessarily action."
—Dr. James O. Prochaska

This chapter will help you get started on your journey to achieve and maintain changes or improvements in a health behavior of most value to you (for example, weight loss, cigarette smoking, and so on) by showing you how to identify your current Stage of Change. Chapter 2 will help you identify and apply processes and techniques that will help you move successfully from your current Stage of Change toward achieving and maintaining your goal. When embarking on the journey of self-change, it is important to accept yourself at whatever stage you are currently in and to accept that change means progress not just action. The Stage of Change model was not intended for anyone to stand in judgment of themselves or others. It was created to understand where one currently is in the change continuum for a particular health behavior, and how to continue to move forward toward permanent change, at one's own pace. Because change can be difficult, it is recommended that you prioritize the behaviors you would like to change, and ideally work on one or two behaviors at a time to maximize success. This approach will allow you to dedicate most of your time, effort, and attention on the behaviors most important to you, without getting overwhelmed and setting yourself up for possible disappointment. Once you have mastered changing your highest priority behavior, you will have gained the confidence and skills that you can then apply to changing other behaviors, if needed, at a later time.

The self-assessment detailed on page 27 will help you identify what Stage of Change you are currently in, for the desired behavior you want to change or improve. By doing so, you will have a clearer understanding of where you are as you begin your journey toward achieving your goal. Chapter 2 will outline and describe the Processes of Change, guiding you to take the appropriate steps toward your goal that are tailored to, or based on, your current Stage of Change.

Often, people struggle with change. In fact, if you are struggling with changing your health behaviors, you are in the majority, not the minority. Research on health behavior change examining adherence to recommendations concerning physical activity, tobacco use, alcohol consumption, fruit and vegetable consumption, and dietary fat intake in U.S. adults discovered that only 6 percent follow all public health recommendations. In addition, nearly 80 percent did not follow health behavior recommendations for these five health behaviors, 42 percent did not adhere to a single recommendation regarding tobacco and/or alcohol, and one or more of the three recommendations regarding diet and exercise (Berrigan, Troiano, Krebs-Smith, and Barbash, 2003). Additional research on health behavior change illustrated that only 20 percent of the population with poor health behaviors are preparing or taking *action* to change them. The remaining 80 percent of the population is in *precontemplation* or *contemplation*. So, again, it's important to note that change does not necessarily mean *action*. You can be making changes in *precontemplation*, such as obtaining more information on your health habits, but not yet acting on them. This is progress; this is change!

It is also important to note that one does *not* progress quickly or linearly through the stages. This does not mean that progress isn't being made at all, but rather that sometimes people may not be ready for *action* and/or face challenges outside of their control. You can be making changes along the way. This can be described as a never-ending game of Chutes and Ladders. Chutes and Ladders is a well-known board game developed by Milton Bradley in 1943 and commercially sold in the United States. Chutes and Ladders has been used as a metaphor for life, and it is also an appropriate metaphor for the Stages of Change. However, instead of leaving your health to the unpredictability of rolling dice, you have the power to act on what you want to change to move up the ladder. Challenges you may face on your journey of change are like the chutes in the game that could bring you back down or impair your progress, but not all chutes are the same length, nor the same setback. Just like each spin of the wheel, so are the *conditions* for change that people are in. Each Stage of Change is detailed below, and entails a series of tasks that need to be completed before progressing to the next stage. It is important to note again that each stage does not inevitably lead to the next Stage of Change. It is possible to get stuck at one stage or spiral up and down to later and earlier stages, respectively, throughout your change process (Prochaska et al., 2002). To achieve and maintain success, first identify the stage you are currently in by completing the following self-assessment, read about your stage, and then focus on the recommended processes in Chapter 2.

Stages of Change Assessment

Keeping in mind the behavior you want to change, which one of the following four statements applies to you?

1. I took action on my health behavior problem more than six months ago.
2. I have taken action on my health behavior problem within the past six months.
3. I am intending to take action on my health behavior problem in the next month.
4. I am intending to take action in the next six months.

Adapted from *Changing for Good* by Prochaska, Norcross, and Di-Clemente (2002).

What stage are you currently in?

- If you answered no to all four statements, you are in *precontemplation*. This means you have no plans to change your health behavior at this time.

- If you answered yes to Question 4, and no to the other three, you are in *contemplation*. You are thinking about or have intentions to taking action on your health behavior problem, but "down the road," not right now. You may still be weighing the pros or benefits of change with the cons or barriers to change.

- If you answer yes to Questions 3 and 4, you are in *preparation*, preparing for action.

- If you answered no to Question 1 and yes to Question 2, you are in *action*, and in the midst of achieving your desired behavior.

- If you answered yes to Question 1, you are in *maintenance* and already taking steps to successfully sustain your changed behavior.

The Stages of Change

The Six Stages of Change include:

1. Precontemplation (not intending on taking action in the foreseeable future).

2. Contemplation (intending to make a change in the future, but not right now).

3. Preparation (intending to take action in the next month).

4. Action (modifying behavior, experiences, or environment in the past six months to make a change).

5. Maintenance (sustaining change for more than six months).

6. Termination (sustaining change for five years or more).

Once you determine what stage you are currently in from this assessment, it is important to accept that you may not actually take action in the time frame you originally planned for yourself. For example, a contemplator could be "stuck" in *contemplation* for years, although his or her original intent was to change in six months. The speed at which you actually move through the stages is individually dependant, as well as how effectively you use the processes outlined in Chapter 2 and other techniques described throughout this book. The Stages of Change can be used to assess, as well as re-assess, your readiness to change the behavior(s) you are currently focusing on, or planning to focus on in the future. Assessing and reassessing your readiness to change will reward you as you make progress and/or help you refocus your efforts during challenging times. It will also assist you in identifying the appropriate "Processes of Change" to employ (Sun, Prochaska, Velicer, and Laforge, 2007). The reason for assessing readiness to change periodically for every behavior is because while you may be taking steps to change one behavior (*action*), you may be in *precontemplation* for another. Periodic

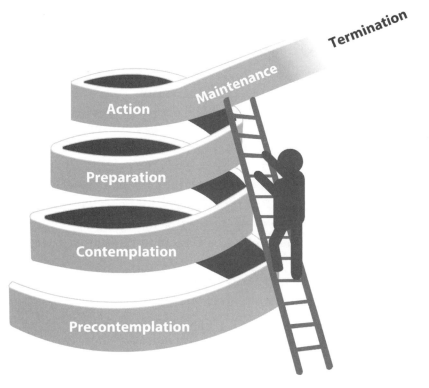

Charles Desper Designs

re-assessment of your Stages of Change will help support and sustain positive and multiple health behavior changes. Research has shown that individuals who try to make changes they are not ready for set themselves up for failure. Also, if one spends too much time working on things he or she has already mastered, such as understanding the "pros" (benefits) and "cons" (challenges) to changing one's current health behavior, he or she may delay acting or moving forward (Prochaska, et al., 2002).

Is my behavior a problem or a preference?

John, a member of my health club, exercised regularly. Although John ate a very poor diet, he was comfortable with his nutritional habits. John frequented fast food restaurants, drank sugar-sweetened beverages in excess, and indulged on candy and desserts throughout the day. He also consumed large portions of food in the evenings. Though I knew his behavior was a problem, John made it clear that he simply preferred to eat this way. John was not defensive about it, nor did he rationalize his eating habits. During our discussion, it became obvious that John was well aware of the health consequences related to these types of eating habits, but it was his preference. I could see John's commitment to improving his physical strength and endurance on a nearly daily basis. As John's health coach, I was confused by John's decision to "undo" the calories he burned by eating this way. But, I respected his decision and continued working with him on the behaviors he was ready to change. I regularly reinforced his physical activity accomplishments, continued "soft nudges" regarding his eating habits, and reinforced that I would make myself available in the future to work on dietary changes with him if, and when, he was ready.

One can tell if his or her behavior is a problem or a preference by honestly answering the following three questions:

1. Do you discuss your health behaviors without becoming defensive?
2. Are you well informed about your health behaviors?
3. Are you willing to take personal responsibility for the consequences of your health behaviors?

If you answer no to one or more of these questions, you are most likely in *precontemplation*. If you answered yes to most of these questions your health behaviors may be a personal preference. If your health behaviors are a personal preference, you may not respond to the recommended courses of action to change. However, over time you may move to *contemplation*, closer to *action*. Chances are, if you are reading this book, some of your health behaviors are not your preference, and you are most likely in the stage of *contemplation*, *preparation*, or *action*. Or, if you are in maintenance, you may be looking for additional support to sustain the positive changes you have already made in your life, or you may be seeking guidance on how to help someone else. Now that you have staged the behavior you want to change, and determined if your behavior is a problem or a preference, read about each stage on the following pages.

Precontemplation

I have consulted for many organizations throughout the years on population (as well as individual) health management. I work with organizations on designing health, wellness, and behavior change strategies for their employees, patients, and/or health plan members. One of my clients, a home healthcare company, was experiencing increasing healthcare and related costs. Like many other clients, they wanted to improve the health of the population as part of the solution to controlling these costs. The home healthcare specialists, predominately nurses, were well educated and trained in the health field. As a population, their claims data and medical expenditures indicated they were very unhealthy. Based on their expertise in healthcare, it was evident they *knew* what to do to get healthy, but they just weren't doing it. It was a revelation for my client. The answer, of course, is they just were not ready to change some of their poor health habits. But as it turned out, they *were* ready to change some.

Smoking was one of the many serious health risks (and cost drivers) in this population, and the most prevalent, so we jointly decided to address that health behavior. I was amazed at how many of the nurses smoked, knowing the dangers of smoking and seeing the results of smoking in the health of their patients on a daily basis. I thought if anyone would know what to do to stay healthy, nurses would. Yet, when we surveyed them, a small percentage indicated they were ready to quit smoking. Most indicated they had no intention of quitting smoking and they would not participate in any programs offered, regardless of any incentives to do so (many employers offer substantial incentives to promote healthy behaviors and/or health outcomes among their employees). It was evident that the majority of this population of home healthcare nurses were in *precontemplation* for quitting smoking. They were just not ready to quit and had no intention of quitting in the near future.

Knowing what stage the majority of the population was in, I could provide more effective, staged-matched, and long-term interventions or program recommendations to move the nurses along the Stages of Change or stage continuum. It would not have been effective to begin recommending adherence to a smoking cessation program (an *action* stage programmatic approach). Because the majority of the nurses were in *precontemplation* for smoking, participation in an *action-oriented* program would have been very low and costly, because the chances of anyone actually quitting would be minimal. Therefore, in collaboration with my client, we decided to focus on a communication campaign, focusing on increasing the "pros" or the benefits of quitting smoking, a "soft-nudge" educational campaign. We coupled this campaign with the launch of a weight-loss program, another problem behavior that was identified within the population. We focused on preparation and action-oriented programs for weight loss, as survey results indicated the population was ready to change this behavior. We had great success with this approach, and an additional benefit that emerged from the campaign coupled with the weight loss program was an increase in readiness to quit smoking! As the nurses' confidence increased from successfully completing weight-loss program, they felt better and were willing to tackle this more difficult behavior of quitting smoking! It was amazing to witness collateral consequences of behavior change! The science supports the phenomena of "coaction," where effective change on one behavior leads to an increase in the probability of change on another behavior (Prochaska, 2008; Johnson et al., 2013).

There are some common characteristics of precontemplators. Denial is one. For example, some alcoholics possess a common denial characteristic of *precontemplation*—not thinking they have a problem. Until active alcoholics face the reality of their behavior and accepts the need to change, they will not move out of *precontemplation*. Individuals with diabetes or other chronic diseases may also be in denial about the cumulative impact of that "one dessert," or not exercising today, tomorrow, or at all. One could deny the damage resulting from not managing one's disease. Individuals may also be in denial that they cannot do anything to help themselves, because they believe their disease is already out of their control. Part of the denial associated with *precontemplation* may be blaming one's poor health on hereditary, societal factors, addiction, or if one feels they have tried everything and nothing has worked. Those are real feelings—real beliefs that are not meant to be judged, but to be dealt with to recognize something *can* be done to improve one's health. The approach may just need to be different, a bit less rigorous, and with a more supportive environment or approach. A "drill sergeant" for a personal trainer may not work for someone in denial. Individuals in denial may respond better to someone who is willing to work *with* them, where they are at in *precontemplation*, helping them move along at their own pace.

Another consideration to be aware of is the possibility of feeling demoralized and helpless while in *precontemplation*. You may have experienced attempting to change several times, been unsuccessful, and said, "Why bother?" It is very important to acknowledge those feelings, and use the processes and techniques in this book to build up your confidence so that you will be successful as you continue your journey toward changing and improving your health. "The good news is that research has demonstrated that even precontemplators can progress toward change if they are given the proper tools at the proper times" (Prochaska et al., 2002, p. 41). I love the commercial for the health club that says it is a "judgment-free zone." This approach is a call out to precontemplators and contemplators.

Common Characteristics of Individuals in Precontemplation

- Not intending to take action in the next six months.
- Denial of problem behavior.
- Blaming problem on hereditary factors, societal factors, or others.
- Feelings of demoralization and hopelessness associated with having "tried everything, but nothing ever works."
- Showing up to programs because of pressure from others such as employers (to qualify for incentives) or partners.

Contemplation

It was about six months after I began working for a global human resources consulting firm as a national subject matter expert in employer health management that I began traveling extensively. Subject matter experts in this area are in high demand across the country as employers struggle with skyrocketing employee healthcare costs. It was terrific to see wellness being recognized as part of the solution for corporations to control these escalating healthcare and productivity costs. As one of the national subject matter experts, I loved the job, and my clients! But, the position required extensive travel, as I was responsible for numerous clients across their North American region. If not managed well, traveling can take its toll on your health, and it did on mine! I gained at least 15 pounds in just my first year on the job. My lifestyle and routines, as I had known and maintained for decades, had changed dramatically to accommodate the demands of the job. I was "up in the air" every week, many weeks traveling to multiple cities across the country and across multiple time zones. My workout routine was totally disrupted. I could not go to my favorite yoga studio and take my regular class with my friends, or exercise on my usual days and at my usual times. Unpredictable and extensive travel basically prohibited me from keeping *any* kind of schedule or routine. My access to healthy food also changed. I couldn't prepare my meals or grocery shop to get the foods I wanted and needed to eat healthy and maintain a healthy weight. I was surrounded by easier and plentiful access to high-caloric food in airports and restaurants. My normal sleeping patterns were also affected. Without a regular and predictable routine, and frequenting hotels, it was also difficult to get regular, quality sleep.

After decades of being in "termination" for weight management, healthy eating, sleep, and exercise, I fell down the "chute" from termination to contemplation. I *knew* I had a problem. I was in the wellness business, for goodness sake! But, I continually made excuses for my unhealthy lifestyle behaviors, and honestly couldn't really see how I could make the necessary changes to return to "action" with my "jet set" lifestyle. I found myself getting on a plane early morning, then off to client meetings all afternoon, then client dinners in the evening, ending with e-mails piled up from the day and having to work late at night. In the end, I felt I had *no* time to maintain a healthy lifestyle and "something had to give." Ironically, it was my health.

One day, after months of *contemplation*, I realized how bad I felt physically and emotionally, and was finally ready to take *action*. I decided to "self-coach" myself using techniques and strategies presented throughout this book. I began my journey by writing down a list of all of my barriers, possible solutions for those barriers, and the Processes of Change that I could leverage (Chapter 2). I began to tackle the list. Slowly but surely, over six months I made it a priority to adjust my work schedule, got a new routine together, and made adaptations necessary to get me back on track and prepare for *action*. I experienced a dramatic change in my lifestyle, as I slowly but surely worked on climbing back up the "ladder" of positive health behavior change.

Do you sometimes clearly see and understand the benefits of change, but other times remind yourself of the many barriers that exist for you to achieve and sustain change? If you answered yes to this question, you are in *contemplation*, but don't get discouraged. Even thinking about changing is progress! Progress may be made at each stage with progression to the next, as we maintain continual commitment to improving our health. It is easy to get "stuck" in contemplation and become a "chronic contemplator." This may be avoided with a continuous commitment to change and by using the Processes of Change. *Contemplation* may be the more difficult state to progress from, but with commitment, many people *can and do* make progress and successfully achieve and maintain their goals.

Common Characteristics of Individuals in Contemplation

- ~ Intending to take action in the next six months.
- ~ Perceived barriers to change outweigh perceived benefits.
- ~ A feeling of being "stuck" that may last for years.
- ~ Telling oneself they will change in the future.
- ~ Rationalization or justification of one's current behavior(s).
- ~ Continuous evaluation of the pros and cons of change.

Preparation

The majority of people who came through the door of my health club to inquire about membership were likely in *preparation*. They were aware of the benefits of change, more conscious of their problem behavior as well as the negative effects of this behavior on their health. Most inquirers did not come in with gym bags or in workout clothes, and were not ready to sign up for an exercise class or workout. They were simply weighing thoughts related to the benefits of membership, preparing for *action*. Some inquirers may have been asking themselves many questions. "Will this be a supportive environment for what I want to accomplish?"

"Can I really commit the necessary time to achieve my goal?" "Can I make the additional commitments needed to achieve my goal (improve my diet, secure child care)?" "Can this personal health trainer even 'relate' to where I am coming from?" These may have just been *some* of the questions the inquirers were tossing around in their minds before making any final commitments to *action*. Inquirers who entered my health club in workout clothes to get prices on membership or to try a free exercise class or workout, were most likely closer to *action*, perhaps ready to begin their journey toward improving their health.

In *preparation*, you may be exploring your exercise options, shopping for a gym to join or exercise equipment, searching for meal plans, or researching smoking cessation programs. Congratulations! You are preparing yourself for change. As you seek information, it is important for you to thoroughly review and evaluate all of the options and resources available to you to support you on your journey of change. Ensure your health resources come from reliable, evidence-based sources. Everything on the Internet is not reliable, so speak with licensed healthcare professionals; obtain health education materials from public and/ or private academic, research, or healthcare institutions whose practices are sound and evidence-based. Of equal importance is to ensure the resources you choose and individuals you work with are a good "fit" for your personality type and the pace at which you are willing and able to work.

Another important part of your success will be dependent on the amount of time you dedicate to *preparation*. The most successful people, who embark on their journey of change, take adequate time in *preparation*. They evaluate all options, making adjustments as needed to position themselves up for success, before they jump into *action*. However, there are exceptions to every rule! For example, my father smoked for nearly two decades. One day, he just quit "cold turkey." Three decades of research supports the likelihood that he would have relapsed based on the fact that he did not adequately "prepare" for this change. But my father was successful against the odds. He not only quit, he quit *permanently*. So, as with any theory or research findings, there are exceptions.

Common Characteristics of Individuals in Preparation

- ๏ Intending to take action in the next month to six months.
- ๏ Taking steps to evaluate options to prepare for change.
- ๏ The pros outweigh the cons of changing.
- ๏ Making final plans and adjustments to current lifestyle.
- ๏ May have already begun to take small steps toward change (for example, cutting back on sweets or smoking fewer cigarettes).

Action

Individuals who are adhering to a regular exercise program, who have made positive dietary changes, who have quit smoking, or who have made any other positive health behavior changes are in *action*. Once in *action*, one is not yet "out of the woods," as he or she must now work toward sustaining change over time. One of the most important issues in the health club industry is member retention. Keeping members in *action* and moving them to *maintenance* is one of the industry's primary goals. However, health clubs struggle to keep members in action and move them to *maintenance*. Health club member dropout rates have been reported to be as high as 50 percent. The *International Health, Racquet and Sportsclub Association (IHRSA)* report a lower dropout rate of 26 percent for their multi-purpose, larger facilities. Although significantly better, more than one out of every four people who join still drop out. The issue of retention to healthy behaviors is not just a problem for the health club industry, but a national issue as well. Many individuals struggle to stay in *action*. According to 2012 statistics published by the University of Scranton, 45 percent of Americans typically make New Year's resolutions. Not surprisingly, the most popular annual resolution of most Americans is to lose weight. However, only 8 percent of individuals achieve their annual weight loss goals (Norcross, Mrykalo, and Blagys, 2002). The same New Year's resolutions are typically made three years in a row before maintenance of behavior change is achieved (Prochaska, et al., 2002). Learning the theories and practicing the strategies and techniques presented in this book is critical for *maintenance*. Although action is a very personally significant accomplishment, it does not automatically translate into *maintenance* or sustained behavior change. More work still needs to be done. Individuals in *action* may successfully progress to *maintenance* or may still be vulnerable to relapse or falling back to the stages of *preparation*, *contemplation*, or even *precontemplation*. Research in the field of health behavior change has shown that the first six months are crucial to determining whether an individual will remain in *action* or revert back to former behaviors (Miller and Hester, 1980). If you are already in *action*, congratulations! The statistics mentioned previously are not intended to discourage you, but to increase your awareness that all of us embarking on the journey of behavior change may be still vulnerable to relapse or lapses in *action*. However, with continual commitment, and increased self-confidence or self-efficacy, positive health behavior changes may be sustained. Your journey does not end at action, but your accomplishment needs to be recognized and applauded!

Common Characteristics of Individuals in Action

- ᴇ Have taken action within the past six months.
- ᴇ Individuals start or stop behaviors they want to change.
- ᴇ Most visible "Stage of Change" observed by others.

Maintenance

"Change never ends with action (Prochaska, et al., 2002)."

Individuals who have been engaging in a health behavior change goal such as increased physical activity, and have successfully done so for a sustained period of time, typically six months or more, are considered to be in *maintenance*. The new behavior of being physically active has replaced a previous sedentary lifestyle, and has been sustained for a significant, and critical, amount of time. However, as with action, continual work is needed to maintain or sustain the progress that has been made through the stage continuum. *Maintenance* is the stage in which individuals work hard to prevent relapsing or reverting back to their old behaviors. Relapse may or may not occur during any Stage of Change. The important thing to note is that if one does relapse, he or she always learns something new that may lead to increased awareness and subsequent sustained behavior change.

Characteristics of Individuals in Maintenance

- ❧ Sustained "action"/new behavior for six months or more.
- ❧ Successful integration of change into one's lifestyle.
- ❧ Successful removal of or overcoming of barriers to maintaining new or changed behavior.
- ❧ Strong commitment to avoiding lapses or relapse.

Termination: The Ultimate Goal of Self-Changers

When Jeff, a member of my health club came in and joined, he was very overweight and was consuming four liters of soda per day! Jeff's lifestyle behaviors were very unhealthy. The first thing I suggested to Jeff was to begin making changes to his lifestyle slowly and steadily at his own pace as I reviewed the processes and techniques presented in this book. Jeff achieved *maintenance* within seven and a half months. Throughout the course several years, Jeff lost 75 pounds, was physically active on a regular basis, and eliminated soda from his diet completely. He had successfully sustained his new behaviors for years without relapse. Jeff was a new person, physically and mentally. When Jeff told me that the thought of drinking all that soda "grossed him out," I knew Jeff had reached *termination*. His new lifestyle was his new "normal." The most rewarding part of being a personal trainer, health coach, or health club owner, is to observe a client "turning the corner" into *maintenance* or *termination* and achieve a permanent healthy lifestyle. Some clients may tell you they no longer crave those late-night potato chip binges, or, in fact, they are turned off by the very idea! Others may tell you that when they skip a workout, they miss it! When I see individuals transform their lives, and go from a sedentary lifestyle and poor eating habits, to enjoying and or even craving their new healthy lifestyle behaviors, it is awesome!

Termination is the ultimate goal of behavior change. *Termination* occurs when one has completed the Stage of Change processes and is no longer working to sustain maintenance of his or her health behavior; it has become the new "norm." However, in most cases, changing behavior is a fluid process in which one moves in and out of the Stages of Change multiple times. *Termination* as a step in behavior change is controversial, as many believe once you have had a problem behavior, you will be in *maintenance* for a lifetime. Take alcoholism, for example. It is believed, once an alcoholic, always an alcoholic. You just take one day at a time to maintain your alcohol-free lifestyle. Others believe one can terminate a problem behavior when one has achieved total confidence in sustaining the new behavior in any and all high-risk situations. In *termination*, one does not feel tempted any longer or feel the threat of relapse. Your ultimate goal is to achieve *termination* of that old behavior! It may take work, and there will be barriers, but you can do it!

Characteristics of Termination

- ๏ Ultimate goal for self-changers.
- ๏ New behavior is the "norm."
- ๏ Old behavior is no longer a temptation or threat under any situation or circumstance.

The following chapters will outline the processes, strategies, and techniques to help move you through the stages to *termination*. As you read this book, and re-evaluate what stage you are in, don't forget that any movement from one stage to another is progress and success! Finally, never forget to give yourself credit and recognition for any and all progress you make on your journey of change.

Key Points

- ๏ The six Stages of Change are *precontemplation, contemplation, preparation, action, maintenance,* and *termination.*
- ๏ "Change means *progress,* not necessarily action."
- ๏ Progression through the stages is not "linear," but movement is in more of a spiral form.
- ๏ Progress is achieved with movement from one stage to the next along the continuum of behavior change.
- ๏ Change does not end with *action.*

- The ultimate goal of positive health behavior change is *termination*.

Action Items

- Complete the Stages of Change Assessment for each behavior you are seeking to change.
- Repeat the Assessment periodically to assess and re-assess your progress.

2

How Do I Start?

Insider Secret #2:
Strategies to Start Changing

As a consultant to a variety of companies and organizations, I develop health-improvement strategies for employee wellness programs. To develop a targeted plan, I first need to review results of the group's health data, including health risk assessments and medical claims of program participants. Often individuals indicate on their self-reported health assessments that their current health is excellent or good. However, upon review of clinical laboratory results or medical claims data, a very different picture emerges. One employer's aggregate data of health assessment results demonstrated 86 percent of participating employees self-reported they were in excellent, very good, or good health. However, the results of biometric screening, or a short health examination that determines one's level of risk for certain diseases and medical conditions, showed that 80 percent of the population was in fact obese or overweight, and more than 60 percent of the population was at risk for both cardiovascular disease *and* diabetes. This huge disparity in the health data is just one example underscoring the importance of raising one's consciousness of current and accurate health status before contemplation of a behavior change is even possible. We may be unaware of our current state of health, as well as how our current lifestyle behaviors may increase our risk for disease. This information was a sign that many of the employees were in *precontemplation*. They had reported that they were completely unaware or uninformed about their true health status. Employing strategies from the Transtheoretical Model of Behavior change (TTM), including the "Processes of Change," such as Consciousness Raising, is an excellent place to begin our journey of change with increased knowledge and self-awareness of our current health status.

Once you have determined your current Stage of Change for the priority health behavior that you are focusing on changing (Chapter 1), you are ready to learn and apply the Processes of Change as you move toward *action* and, ultimately, *maintenance*. There are 10 Processes of Change that are "covert and overt activities that people use to progress through the stages" (Prochaska and Velicer, 1997, p. 39). To progress through the early stages, people apply cognitive, affective, and evaluative processes. As people move toward *action* and *maintenance*, they rely more on commitments, conditioning, contingencies, environmental controls, and support (Prochaska, Redding, and Evers, 2002). Prochaska and colleagues state that their research related to TTM shows that interventions to change behavior are more effective if they are "stage-matched," or "matched to each individual's stage of change." The 10 Processes of Change are essentially a combination of a variety of evidence-based behavior change theories and techniques to maximize your success as you move through the Stages of Change. Per Dr. James Prochaska, one must consider the "What, When, How, Pros, Who, and Where" of health behavior change as listed here:

- The What: The behavior you desire to change.
- The When: The Stage of Change.
- The How: The Processes of Change.
- The Pros: The Whys.
- The Who: You.
- The Where: Anywhere.

The Stages of Change will reveal *what* Stage of Change you are in, whereas the Processes of Change show you *how* you can move through the continuum of change. The Processes of Change are like "tools" in a toolbox that we can take and use with us on our journey toward change. You can leverage one or all of these "tools," depending upon individual needs at a particular point in time. These processes have been successfully and effectively used for more than three decades and are based on sound research. It is important to note that you can start using the processes even if you are not ready for action.

The 10 Processes of Change include:

- ᴥ Consciousness Raising: Become aware, educated, and informed.
- ᴥ Environmental Reevaluation: Consider the effect on others.
- ᴥ Dramatic Relief: Increase emotional arousal and reaction to the need to change.
- ᴥ Social Liberation: Leverage public supports, opportunities, and resources.
- ᴥ Self-Reevaluation: Clarify what you need or want to change (now emotionally vested).
- ᴥ Self-Liberation: "Commit to it and stick to it."
- ᴥ Helping Relationships: Rally your support "troops," to include friends, family, and colleagues.
- ᴥ Counterconditioning: Develop substitutes for unhealthy behaviors.
- ᴥ Stimulus Control: Adjust your environment to support your change.
- ᴥ Reinforcement Management: Reward and recognize your progress.

The 10 Processes of Change best used at each Stage of Change is shown and described in detail as follows (Prochaska and Velicer, 1997):

Precontemplation	Contemplation	Preparation	Action	Maintenance
Consciousness Raising				
Environmental Reevaluation				
Dramatic Relief				
Social Liberation				
	Self Reevaluation			
		Self-Liberation		
		Helping Relationships		
		Counter Conditioning		
			Stimulus Control	
			Reinforcement Management	

Consciousness Raising

Consciousness Raising occurs when we exert efforts to seek out new information and attempt to heighten awareness of ourselves and our problem behavior. This process was first described by Sigmund Freud, who said the basic objective was to "make the unconscious conscious (Prochaska *et al.*, 2002)." The goal of this process is to increase your level of awareness of both yourself *and* your health behavior. This may sound simple, yet it can be difficult. Have you ever heard your voice on tape, or saw a picture of yourself and said, "Is that really me?" To varying degrees, we may all be somewhat unconscious of our true self, our true behaviors, and the effect on our health and on others. We also may need to increase our consciousness of our behavior, its effects, and what is actually required of us to make progress and for change to actually take place.

When I served as the director of the governor of Rhode Island's wellness initiative, *Get Fit, Rhode Island*, I led more than 25 extraordinary "Wellness Champions," representing each department of state government. The Champions were appointed by their respective department director and possessed an uncanny ability to inspire others to engage in or increase healthy behaviors. The Champions were, in essence, the "wellness influencers" or change agents within their departments. To promote increased physical activity among state employees working in the Rhode Island State House and its surrounding departments, Sue Stenhouse, the State House Wellness Champion, mapped out an indoor walking route within the State House.

The route, covering three levels and utilizing the marble stairwells, was around 2,000 steps in length, a walk that could be accomplished by employees during lunchtime. Sue also made this initiative interesting, as it was a historical walk through one of the most beautiful structures in Rhode Island. In fact, the dome of the Rhode State House is the fourth-largest self-supporting marble dome in the world, after St. Peter's Basilica, the Minnesota State Capitol, and the Taj Mahal. Tom, an employee seeking to lose weight, heard about the walk from another state department, but said he could not join the walking group because he simply felt he was "too out of shape." He did not believe he could walk the 2,000 steps. Sue helped raise her colleague's "consciousness" about how much walking was required to be beneficial. Sue explained to Tom that it was still beneficial for him to walk across the street from his department to the State House, and also beneficial for him to simply walk through the first hallway of the State House and then back to his department.

After a few months of providing information, raising Tom's consciousness, and providing encouragement, Sue got Tom to come over and just "give it a try." Sue walked by his side for encouragement and to monitor his pace. She explained to Tom the philosophy of *Get Fit, Rhode Island*: Some exercise was better than no exercise at all. My Wellness Champions and I continuously promoted the finding of current research with our state employees. In this case, we explained to Tom that three, 10-minute bouts of exercise in the same day resulted in the same health benefits as one continuous bout of 30 minutes of exercise (Foulds, Bredin, Charlesworth, Ivey, and Warburton, 2014).

We raised the awareness of our employees who now knew that many of hours of sitting on a daily basis, or a sedentary lifestyle, is a risk factor for obesity and its many related chronic diseases. By the simple nature of their jobs, many state employees sat at their desks and computers most of the day. Collectively, my Wellness Champions and I set out to increase our employees' knowledge, raising their consciousness of the amount *and* spacing of exercise that would be beneficial to them. With "raised consciousness" of this new information, some employees like Tom moved up the change continuum. We were proud that many employees who would not have participated were now interested and involved after this new knowledge. Tom's ultimate engagement in the State House walk was a true testament to the success of the *Get Fit* program.

> *"Knowledge is POWER!"*
> —Francis Bacon

The more you increase your knowledge and consciousness of the behavior you are seeking to change, the more likely you will be to move toward, make, and sustain the change. Consciousness Raising is most beneficial for those in *precontemplation* or *contemplation*. If you find yourself saying *"I want to change, BUT...,"* this process is for you! To raise consciousness of the behavior you want to change is to also increase knowledge about yourself and to be fully aware of how your problem behavior is affecting your health and others. This can be difficult for an individual in denial. But awareness of denial can also raise consciousness. When we accept that we may be in denial or rationalizing a particular behavior, we move forward toward *preparation* and *action* when we are ready.

Tips for Consciousness Raising

- ↝ Subscribe to a reputable and credible health magazine based on new and current evidence-based research and begin to read about your problem behavior.

- ↝ Seek information from licensed health care professionals such as your doctor.

- ↝ Make a relaxing visit to a bookstore and browse through books and health magazines on the behavior you would like to change.

- ↝ Read blogs and/or follow subject matter experts on social networking sites; follow me on Twitter @annieludovici or visit my Website (*www.annemarieludovici.com*) for updated information to help you change.

- ↝ Recall: Think back on information people may have provided in the past about how to change your behavior. You may not have been ready to hear it at the time, but may now be ready to process the information.

- ↝ Ask others who have succeeded to share their stories and listen for ways you may be able to model their behaviors.

- ↝ Ask people closest to you to be honest about your behavior.

Sometimes precontemplators do not want to ask their doctors or those closest to them about their problem behavior or the effects their behavior may be having on their health, simply because they do not want to know. This is natural. However, one does not have to be *ready* for *action* while gathering this information. The purposes of this process are to raise consciousness and awareness about a problem behavior and begin making progress. Gathering facts and keeping them in a "quiver" will help facilitate action if and when one is ready.

Environmental Reevaluation

Environmental Reevaluation is when we realize, consider, and evaluate how our problem behavior affects those around us or the physical environment. Debbie smoked for more than 10 years and was not thinking about quitting. However, she came across an article and was reminded of the negative effects of secondhand smoke on others. With this "reminder," Debbie began to think of her son and the relatives who now lived with her. She was horrified when she finally came to realize that her family's health was also at risk because of her smoking. Debbie began to reassess and reconsider her smoking behavior. Debbie was single and also considered how her smoking was negatively affecting her social life. Debbie was dating, as well going out with her friends. Most of them didn't smoke and disliked Debbie's habit. In light of all of these factors, Debbie began to move toward *preparation* by asking her doctor and her health plan for information to begin to discover options, and the best way for her to quit smoking. Debbie was moving closer to *action* through this process of change.

Tips for Environmental Reevaluation

- Learn about how your health behaviors affect others and the environment.
- Think about who in your life may be positively or negatively affected by your health behaviors.

Dramatic Relief

Dramatic Relief is experiencing strong emotions or feels, an enlightenment of sorts, about our problem behavior along with a discovery of possible solutions. At an event to celebrate an award given to *Get Fit, Rhode Island*, a state employee, Charlene, gave a powerful testimony about her personal health transformation. Charlene shared how *Get Fit* "saved her life." At a health screening event offered at work, Charlene found out she was on the verge of having a cardiac event. As Charlene told her story and shared intimate details about her health and her young family, she became very emotional. As I looked around the room, I observed the eyes of the audience glued to her. The room was silent as the attendees hung on her every word. It appeared that everyone was captivated by Charlene's story, which aroused emotions at a core and visceral level. Later, some attendees shared that they related to Charlene's story and were so inspired that it helped them initiate their own healthy behavior changes. Charlene's dramatic testimony "nudged" individuals in the audience who were not previously ready to commence their own journeys of change.

Individuals may experience emotional arousal when a friend or family member is diagnosed with a chronic disease such as heart disease or diabetes. Sometimes it takes a doctor or a loved one to tell us "your health is being seriously compromised" to get our attention. Or perhaps we "hit rock bottom," realizing that our health, and possibly personal relationships, may be in serious jeopardy if we don't change.

Films or movies may also trigger emotional arousal. In the late 1980s, on our annual trip to New York City on Christmas Eve, my late husband, Mark, and I kept our annual tradition of stopping at a well-known national fast food chain to grab a "big burger" for the road. However, after seeing the movie *Supersize Me*, I no longer had the desire to eat burgers from fast-food chains. Emotional arousal may be an extremely powerful force in behavior change by allowing us to deeply connect with our feelings.

Tips for Dramatic Relief

- Read success stories and testimonials. They will help you move along the change continuum.

- Visit your doctor regularly to ensure your preventive health screenings are up to date and you have your most updated results. Ignorance is *not* bliss when it comes to your health. Your current health screening results will help you focus and/or readjust any needed efforts on your journey toward improving your health behaviors.

- Watch a reliable and credible film, *YouTube* video, or commercial on the behavior you want to change.

Social Liberation

Social Liberation is gaining an awareness and acceptance of available resources, policies, social groups, and other alternatives that can support our desired behavior change. Whether they are people, social groups, support groups, organizations, and/or institutional policies (for example, smoke-free), our external environments and support systems may provide us with positive "nudges" toward change. Another benefit of the lunch time walking initiative of *Get Fit* was the social and environmental supports it provided to employees in early Stages of Change. Joining a social group or organization of individuals with common goals will help you move closer to change. Physical changes to environments such as a marked walking route, enticing improvements or renovations to promote use of stairwells versus elevators, installation of bike racks, and healthy food options in cafeterias and vending machines are just some examples of environmental supports for precontemplators and contemplators to achieve positive health behavior change. Organizational policies such as no-smoking policies or policies regarding the nutritional value of foods served onsite or at special events have been proven to promote positive health behavior change. In 2005, the U.S. Centers for Disease Control and Prevention (CDC) reported 20 percent of U.S. adults smoked. That rate has declined to 18 percent, due in large part to the national impact of policy and environmental changes, including smoke-free buildings and workplaces and taxation on tobacco products.

Tips for Social Liberation

- Leverage the improvements to your environment, including stairwell prompts, community walking paths, or healthy menu selections in restaurants.
- Select eating establishments or vacation destinations that have healthy food options, opportunities for physical activity, and so on.
- Research organizations or groups that can help support your change.
- Support or get active in your community to make changes to environments or institute policies in worksites, schools, or child care settings to promote and sustain healthy behavior changes.

Self-Reevaluation

Self-Reevaluation occurs when we reach a rational and emotional reappraisal of our problem behavior and come to the realization of how it aligns with our core values and goals.

Lyrics from The Jimmy Cliff song "I Can See Clearly Now" describe this process well. During Self-Reevaluation, you can now see all the obstacles, or barriers, in your way. And, it's like raising the "dark clouds" that may have had you blind. You are now on your way to a "bright, bright sunshiny" day!

Using the self-assessment in Chapter 1, thoughtfully and reflectively reevaluate your current Stage of Change or readiness to change. Self-Reevaluation will raise your consciousness to the next level. You are now beginning to become very aware of your health status and it is becoming clear that you need to change or continue your progress through the change continuum. Self-Reevaluation keeps your journey illuminated. The more candles you light and keep lit on your journey, the more closely you will be aware of and in touch with your feelings about your health and any necessary actions or readjustments that you need to make. Self-Reevaluation "re-enlightens" you.

Tips for Self-Reevaluation

- ❧ Look at yourself clearly in front of a mirror. Honestly ask yourself, "Is my behavior a problem?"
- ❧ Never stop seeking the truth within yourself. Journaling may be a powerful aid to help you seek and uncover the truth.

Self-Liberation

"There is a difference between interest and commitment. When you are interested in doing something, you do it only when it's convenient. When you're committed to something, you accept no excuses—only results."
—Ken Blanchard

Self-Liberation occurs when we consciously making the choice and commitment to change a problem behavior, and now possess a strong belief in the ability to change. We have moved from an interest in doing (changing) something to a commitment where we accept no excuses—only results, as Ken Blanchard says in the quote. This is a critical process in behavior mastery in order to move to action and sustain later stages of change. I have worked with hundreds of health and wellness vendors who offer their programs through competitions, technology and applications, online modules, and other channels. At the launch of their programs, participants typically sign a "contract" as a way to "cement" their commitment to the program. I have consulted for some workplaces where employees post their contracts on their office doors as a visual reminder of their commitment to themselves, and for their colleagues to witness. Self-Liberation, or making a commitment to yourself and taking self-responsibility, is a critical Process of Change. "Going public" with your commitment improves the efficacy of this process.

Tips for Self-Liberation

- Create and sign a "contract" to adhere to a program. (A sample follows.) Have a backup plan for in the event that you are distracted from your goal by "something that comes up."
- Post your contract on your refrigerator, bedroom mirror, in your car, or at work. Post in multiple places as a visual reminder.
- Commit to attend a regular exercise class with a friend.
- Tell everyone you know about your commitment to maximize your support.
- "Accept no excuses—only results."

> *"If you want to change for good, commit to it and stick to it.*
> *It's easier said than done, but it's as simple as that."*
> —Annie

Sample Contract

> *I,   agree to commit to completing this exercise class, and attend, at a minimum, at least three times per week, for 10 weeks. If something "comes up" and I miss the exercise class, I agree to do my exercise video as a substitute. I will "accept no accuses—only results."*
>
> *Signed:*
> *Witnessed:*
> *Date:*

Helping Relationships

Helping Relationships is when we identify, leverage, and accept help from trusting, accepting, and nurturing relationships throughout our attempts to change a problem behavior.

> *"No one can change a person...but someone can be a person's reason to change."*
> —SpongeBob SquarePants

I have survived some very dark times in my life. I discuss them throughout this book to share the challenges I faced, the lessons I learned, and how even a "wellness expert" can struggle with attaining and maintaining positive health behavior changes, especially during difficult lifecycle changes. One of the darkest periods in my life was my husband's long battle with leukemia and ultimate death. Mark Connolly, my husband and the father of my son, was only 36 years old when his battle ended. I found myself a widow at 33 years of age and a single mother of our 4-year-old son, Kyle. I was completely devastated. I would have never been able to maintain positive health behaviors without my supportive relationships with family, close friends, and neighbors, all reaching out to help me with many things so I could continue to keep my mental and physical health in check. Kyle also fueled the fire I needed to maintain my health. As his mother, I knew I had to stay healthy for him, the most precious person in the world to me. The bottom line was I could not be the mother Kyle needed and deserved at 4 years old if I did not take care of my health. My social supports and Kyle encouraged me to maintain healthy behaviors during a time when I could have easily fallen into a long-term depression. I had to redefine my "new normal." I had to keep going on my journey of health behavior change, mentally and physically, and my journey of life with the help and support of others.

Tips for Helping Relationships

- ❧ Identify people in your life who can provide you with helping relationships and what they may be able to assist you with.
- ❧ Identify specific tasks each of these people can do for you.
- ❧ Don't be afraid to ask for *and* accept help.

- Join support groups and take classes. Weight-loss groups or gyms can provide you with Helping Relationships. Many people in these groups are trying to achieve similar goals, and there is staff to help you as well.
- Leverage the help of experts such as your physician, other healthcare professionals, or health coaches and personal trainers.

Journal Activity

- Make a list of possible Helping Relationships.
- Make a list of your needs and how each relationship may be able to support you.
- Communicate with your team of helpers.

Counterconditioning

Counterconditioning is when we work to identify and discover substitutes or alternatives as a replacement for a problem behavior. When I was caring for my late husband, Mark, throughout his battle with cancer, I was home most of the time and I was extremely stressed. In the evenings, after long and difficult days, I found myself looking for something in the house to eat for emotional comfort. As soon as I realized this impulsive behavior was becoming a problem, I "countered" the behavior of comfort eating with a taking a hot bath or shower. A hot shower or bath between 96 and 105 degrees Fahrenheit, for 10 minutes, has been said to act like a natural sedative, and reduce stress and improve mood in healthy individuals.

Counterconditioning really helped me slow down my weight gain during one of the most stressful times of my life. Learn how to countercondition or substitute a healthy behavior for an unhealthy one. For example, if find yourself stressed and want to binge eat or eat high caloric "comfort foods," you may counter this impulse with a hot shower, calling a close friend, or going for a walk.

Tips for Counterconditioning

- Take a warm shower or bath.
- Do six squats in place.

- ❧ Call a close friend.
- ❧ Take a walk, even if it is just around the outside of your home.
- ❧ Do stretching or yoga exercises.
- ❧ On a nice sunny day, go outside, put your face up to the sun and take deep cleansing breaths.
- ❧ Listen to your favorite music or band.
- ❧ Go for a drive by one of your favorite, peaceful locations.
- ❧ Work on a puzzle.
- ❧ Read a magazine or watch a movie.

Journal Activity

- ❧ Make your list of healthy substitute alternatives.

Stimulus Control

Stimulus Control is when we take control or change the environment or situations, such as adding or remove stimuli or things, which may trigger problem behaviors. In addition, controlling stimuli may encourage alternative improved behaviors.

Sharon, the Wellness Champion for the Rhode Island Department of Administration, worked in the budget division. Her department, like many departments and organizations, was often under tight deadlines. To manage her stress in the wake of a high-performing department, Sharon designed her cubicle to be "Zen-like." Sharon placed a table next to her desk that had a soothing waterfall and a flameless candle. She used aromatherapy oils and displayed seashells she had collected from various beaches in her work area. Sharon practiced chair yoga and deep breathing throughout her workday because she could not take adequate breaks, never mind a full lunch hour.

Tips for Stimulus Control

General

- ❧ Remove any temptations from your environment or anything that can slow your progress (for example, sweets, cigarettes, or alcohol).

- Redesign your home or work environment to reduce distractions from your commitment to change and help manage any stress.

Physical Activity

- Make a workstation exercise basket to include hand weights, a jump rope, and a yoga mat.
- Purchase exercise equipment to *use* in your home or office.

Healthy Eating

- Remove and do not purchase foods that can derail your attempts to improve your eating habits.
- Stock up on healthy foods and snacks so you don't run out.
- Purchase food storage containers, bags, and/or coolers to transport your healthy foods and snacks wherever you go.

Journal Activity

- List the behavior(s) you want to change.
- List ways you can control external stimuli and situations to support your change.

Reinforcement Management

Reinforcement Management occurs when we reward ourselves, or are rewarded by others for making changes. A trend in employer health management or workplace wellness is the use of incentives to drive employee health program participation and improve health outcomes. Employees are rewarded by completing certain health and wellness programs or by achieving certain health outcomes, such as improved body weight, blood pressure, or fasting blood results. Perhaps your employer is offering some type of incentive program. If so, participate if you are in *preparation*, *action*, or *maintenance* for immediate rewards. Rewards have been shown to move people along the continuum of change. Although rewards have not been proven to be as effective in earlier Stages of Change such as *precontemplation* or *contemplation*, they have been shown to increase participation. Paul, a medical professional in a large hospital system, called a health coach to qualify for a financial incentive that his employer was offering. However, Paul refused to discuss changing any of his health behaviors even though most of his clinical laboratory results showed that he was at high risk for metabolic syndrome, a group of risk factors that raises one's risk for heart disease and other health problems, such as diabetes and stroke. Paul said he *knew* his sedentary lifestyle and nutrition behaviors were affecting his health. Paul was a medical professional, highly educated in science and biology. Although Paul was very proud of his education and knowledge of what he *should* be doing, Paul himself was not ready to change. Because Paul was in *precontemplation*, he did not respond as positively to the financial incentives for participating in a health program as he might have if he was in *preparation*, *action*, or *maintenance*. For those in earlier Stages of Change, reinforcement of behavior change may not likely be effective.

Recognition is also a way to promote change. For example, if you have been successful at weight loss, submit your testimonial to a magazine or to the director of your employer's wellness program. Recognition will drive you to maintain your healthy behavior. Complete a walk, run, or bike-a-thon for health and receive a certificate of completion to post as a reminder of your achievement. Recognition and rewards from yourself or others will reinforce the positive behavior change you have made.

Tips for Reinforcement, Rewards, and Recognition

- Participate in a health rewards program at work (if your employer offers one).

- Visibly post or display any current or past certificates of completion or awards for healthy achievements, including medals or trophies from your childhood. (I keep my figure skating and aerobics instructor medals visible to reinforce my current commitment to being physical active and helping others to be physically active as well.)

- Create your own certificate once you complete your health goal. There are various templates available online.

- Write a personal testimonial to recognize yourself for your progress and achievements. Even if no one else sees it, write it for yourself.

- Create your own healthy rewards program. For example, if you adhere to the contract you made with yourself, treat yourself to something related to a healthy hobby, such as fishing lures, a new swimsuit, aromatherapy bath oils, or a massage, keeping within your budget.

Journal Activity

- Make a list of change milestones and possible reinforcements or rewards.

Decisional Balance

Decisional Balance is another component of the Transtheoretical Model that can help identify Stage of Change, but also help move individuals toward later Stages of Change. Decisional Balance is measured by weighing the *pros* or benefits of changing our behavior against the *cons* or costs of changing. In earlier Stages of Change, the cons of changing outweigh the pros. In later Stages of Change, the pros of changing outweigh the cons. Research has shown that we base our decisions to change our health behaviors, in part, on the *pros* and *cons* of doing so. Performing an exercise to measure your Decisional Balance or assess the pros versus cons of change will help you determine the motivational forces behind a problem behavior. You may begin to assess the pros and cons of any behavior change by answering the following four basic questions (adapted from "Changing for Good" by Prochaska, Norcross, and DiClemente, 2002):

1. What are the consequences of change to you?
2. What are the consequences of change to others?
3. How will you react as a result of change?
4. How will others react as a result of change?

Journal Activity

Perform the Decisional Balance exercise by answering the four questions, and writing down the pros and cons for each question. Keep adding to and reflecting on your list over time.

Key Points

- ⚬ The Transtheoretical Model includes 10 Processes of Change.

- ⚬ The Stages of Change will reveal *what* Stage of Change you are in, whereas the Processes of Change show you *how* you can move through the continuum of change.

- ⚬ The Processes of Change are like "tools" in a toolbox. You can leverage one, or all of these "tools," depending upon your needs, and what will work for you, at a particular point in time.

- ⚬ Different Processes of Change have been proven to be more effective at different Stages of Change.

Action Items

- ⚬ Identify the Processes of Change that match your current Stage of Change.

- ⚬ Complete the journal activities to utilize the processes.

- ⚬ Check out Pro-Change Behavior Systems' online behavior change modules for additional support for your lifestyle changes (*www.prochange.com/my health* or *www.prochange. com behavior change-products*).

3

Return to Recess

Insider Secret #3:
Give It a Break and Have Fun!

Recess. The word instantly takes me back to fourth grade. My eyes light up and my smile widens at the very thought of it! The very mention of it to the audiences I address at health and wellness conferences elicit a visceral response. Recess: that fun, social time of the school day when you were free to run, be outdoors, socialize with your friends, and get a break from your studies. Throughout my 30 years in the health and wellness industry, I observed that when people are having *fun* with the new changes they are attempting to make, whether that is increased physical activity, healthier eating, or stress reduction, they were more successful at maintaining or sustaining change. Think of the health change that you are trying to make as recess, or time that you enjoy and look forward to. "Return to Recess." The objective is that the activities you engage in to reach your goal should be something you *want* to do, as opposed to something you *have* to do. When you achieve this mindset, you will have a greater chance of achieving and maintaining your health behavior change.

The difficult part may be finding those activities that you will truly have fun doing. In this chapter, you will learn to find ways that appeal to you on your journey of change, so you can have fun and Return to Recess while doing them. When you Return to Recess you *do not* have to be in the *action* stage of changing your health behavior. You do not have to begin adhering to any physical activity regimen or nutrition guidelines or any other health recommendations to enjoy recess. You may be in *any* stage of change. Earlier in my career, in the 1990s, I worked as a fitness consultant for Club Med Resorts. I worked with guests and staff trained in group physical activity and set up fitness centers at various resorts in Florida and the Caribbean. I was stunned at the amount of individuals, on vacation, who would participate in the various physical activities offered throughout the day. If I assessed what stages of change people were in as they arrived, most would likely be in *precontemplation* or *contemplation* stage. However, Club Med got vacationers to get up and move. Why? Because they made it fun! There were no expectations for physical activity frequency, intensity, or duration. Club Med was almost like a "summer camp" for adults, creating a fun, social, relaxing atmosphere that encouraged people to be physically active. People were relaxed and met others as they got active. Club Med created a positive, uplifting atmosphere so people were in a good mood. The activities were led by energetic, inspiring Gracious Organizers, or "GOs." All of these and other successful elements were woven into Club Med's "secret sauce" of guest engagement. This chapter will describe changes that anyone can make to their home environment to create an atmosphere that supports positive health behavior change so that it becomes a fun, not a dreaded, experience.

As I worked in fitness centers at various Club Med resorts, I had many "weekend warriors" (individuals who are active on weekends but sedentary during the week) ask me for healthy eating and fitness advice. One of our guests, Charlie, was an overweight gentleman who did not engage in regular physical activity at home. Charlie asked me what type of physical activity was best for him to help lose weight once he left the Club. I was excited by the fact that his vacation may have actually inspired him to engage in regular physical activity when he returned home. Imagine that! Can vacation, or taking a break from the grind of daily life, inspire you or change your mind to change your health? The positive lifestyle changes we make in our lives, easier to do without the pressures of the daily grind, can also be maintained when our reality returns and life gets in the way. Strategies for overcoming the barriers to maintaining positive behavior change will be discussed in later chapters. For now, back to Charlie. So, I gave serious thought to Charlie's question, which I am frequently asked as an exercise physiologist. My response was and continues to be the same to this very day: "Whatever you find fun and you will stick with on a regular basis."

This answer tends to annoy some people. It is as though they are expecting a secret, a trick recipe for instant success, something unique, complex, and almost magical. But there is nothing magical about it. Physical activity, or any other positive health behavior, only works if you do it and do it regularly. Research has even proven that the best chance for regular physical activity occurs when the chosen activity has a high satisfaction rate (Fleig, Lippke, Pomp, and Schwarzer, 2011). You will do it when you like it and when it's fun! It is that simple.

Of course, I am not minimizing the importance of physical activity recommendations, dietary guidelines, or any other evidence-based health recommendations, but the fact is, you can still adhere to the guidelines *and* have fun! If we change our mindset we can more easily get physically active or embark on any health behavior change that we have set as our goal. First adhere to the fun, then to the guidelines. As a health club owner, I would tell my instructors and trainers, "If it isn't fun, they aren't going to come." So, I trained my staff to be "educated entertainers." They made every effort to not only ensure members were getting the expert advice needed to achieve their goals, but that they were enjoying themselves in the entire health club experience. The "regulars" who routinely came to work out really had a good time at the club. They enthusiastically participated in the physical activity classes or frequently smiled during their workouts with other members and staff. To be successful at achieving your health goal and to keep motivated, you must love, or learn to love, the physical activity, healthier foods, or other alternative and positive health behaviors you choose to engage in. Of course, the professional health recommendations and guidelines will produce optimal results when followed. They are the "gold standards." However, if not already, you can become a good "matchmaker" by discovering your healthy options for behavior change. You may experience "love at first sight" or you may grow to love the change you have made over time. This chapter will help you do just that.

In my first book, *Winning Health Promotion Strategies* (2010), I share an experience I had when I consulted for Club Med Resorts, an experience worth repeating: "From the moment you open the glossy, enticing travel brochure, to the time you enter the stately wrought iron gates, you are instantaneously attracted. Within a very short period of time, you become completely engaged and entrenched in the culture you have entered into until you exit the resort. The culture may remain a part of you for weeks, and in some cases, months after departure. In my case, it never vacated."

Club Med, whose tagline once was "the antidote for civilization," knows exactly how to attract, engage, and sustain their guests' interests and attention all too well! They not only know how to attract guests seeking to "escape from civilization" by providing a variety of effective, relaxing "antidotes," they know how to engage their guests in daily physical activity—and on vacation to boot! "Everything I learned about motivating people to engage in physical activity, I learned at Club Med!" I have shared this with many diverse audiences at business conferences where I have presented, as well as to many college classes I have taught. This statement may be perceived as an exaggeration, but it does hold merit. Let me explain why. Early in my career, I had the pleasure of working for Club Med in the French Caribbean for a short period of time. I was so excited, as I would not have had the opportunity to visit the French Caribbean otherwise. I was assigned to a few different locations to train Gracious Organizers, or "GOs," on how to effectively teach physical activity classes, and to assist with setting up on-site fitness centers. Some guests declared to me they had not been physically active for many years, yet they kept active daily at Club Med! "What is going on here?" I asked myself. I began to pay attention to what Club Med GOs were doing, and after a few days I got it! I began learning from *their* lead!

Here is my story. When I arrived at Club Med in Guadalupe, I was fresh out of college, and a newly certified health fitness instructor. I knew all the proper protocols for delivering individualized, safe, and effective physical activity prescriptions. I was brought to the location on the property where I was to instruct the physical activity class and train the GO. When I got to the location, I was horrified! I immediately went to Jerome, the "Chef de Village" (French title for "resort manager") and declared "This location is unacceptable!" It was on the beach. I was concerned about floor surface, or lack of, with steep slopes and uneven surfaces on which someone could easily twist an ankle. I was concerned about the blazing sun of the Caribbean, which could lead to dehydration while exercising. I was concerned about improper footwear, as people on the beach did not have shoes on, nor much else for that matter (a story for another day). But, before I could verbalize all of my concerns, Jerome quickly cut me off.

"Oh Onnie (Annie)," Jerome pleasantly said in his French accent. "No problem. No problem, Onnie. Just have FUN!" What? *He is totally blowing me off*, I thought! And, why did everyone always say, "No problem!" This location was a problem. I was certain of it. These conditions could result in injuries! I felt Jerome was patronizing me. Why didn't he get it? But, I returned to the beach where my protégé, Pierre, was waiting for me. Pierre was not well versed in English, and I was not well versed in French. So, on top of every other barrier, Pierre and I had a communication barrier! "This just keeps getting better and better!" I sarcastically said to myself.

Pierre signaled for someone to start the music. It blared from a pair of very large speakers that were perched up high on stands facing the ocean and hidden among the palm trees. I requested that the music be turned down so that guests could clearly hear my instructions. My request was granted. I began the class with about a half dozen people. I was leading the class while showing Pierre how a safe and effective physical activity class should be conducted. After a few minutes, Pierre disappeared. Shortly after I noticed his absence, the music volume was turned up again! I looked down the beach and spotted Pierre. He was gathering guests like the Pied Piper while gyrating to the loud music in his leopard-skin Speedo! He then proceeded to walk back to the class with a large crowd of people in tow! Beach chairs were emptying as most everyone was joining in the class, dancing, moving, and laughing. No one was following my instructions. No one could hear them. No one seemed to care. But everyone was having a blast!

Throughout my time at Club Med, Pierre and I learned how to strike a balance between safe and effective physical activity instruction, and entertaining, engaging instruction. By his lead, Pierre taught me how to meet people *where they wanted to be* (on the beach) and *doing what they wanted to do* (moving to their own beat). And it worked! I taught Pierre how to adapt workouts to the environment and we adapted by avoiding lateral movements in the sand, which, in turn, avoided potential ankle sprains. We taught half the class in the water to address improper footwear and hydration concerns. And we gave water breaks. Although it is sometimes difficult to strike a perfect balance between safety and engagement, I learned that it *is* possible. Now, to this day, in "challenging" physical activity situations, I just think of Pierre and say, "No problem!"

I shared this story to demonstrate the importance of consciously creating an engaging environment and culture for your own wellness journey while avoiding "pasteurizing" wellness. Engagement in wellness is both an art *and* science (Ludovici-Connolly, 2010). As mentioned earlier, studies have shown that when people are enjoying their fitness programs, they regularly adhere to or keep to them. In a large study performed in a workplace setting, one of 10 critical program criteria identified for producing increased participation along with positive outcomes was…FUN! So, how do you begin to discover or *rediscover* activities that you find fun and engaging and want to take the time to do? A good start is to complete an Activity History.

Activity History

Early in my career, I worked for a premier fitness management company, Healthtrax, which now has 18 medical fitness centers throughout the United States. Healthtrax developed an Activity History to be used in initial consultations with new members. In reviewing the Activity History, the fitness trainer asks new members what they currently do for exercise, or to recall a time when they did exercise, and what they liked and disliked about it. The trainer would then probe deeper and ask if the member could exercise again now, what they would change, and how they could augment their previous exercise or physical activity with a new activity. The Activity History is a very effective tool to identify new members' likes and dislikes, to build on past activities, and to help new members discover new activities. Bob Stauble, cofounder and chief administrative officer of Healthtrax, states that the Activity History is one way to help members reach an "Inflection Point," a point at which behavior modification occurs.

Basically, an Activity History is a physical activity recall that helps you think back on activities that you may have performed in your past.

Some of these activities you may have temporarily forgotten about or just became too busy to continue. An Activity History can also improve your confidence by strengthening your "Mastery Experience" (Chapter 4) by recalling the success you had adhering to a specific type or form of physical activity in the past.

I continued utilizing this effective tool when I owned my health club, as I saw how critical it was to member engagement. As part of the initial consultation with new or prospective members, we requested each new member to complete an Activity History before developing a "physical activity prescription" or an individualized physical activity plan. One part of the prescription was based on physical activity guidelines and recommendations, and the other part was based on the new member's Activity History and Stage of Change, and what the new member thought they would enjoy. I would ask new members to tell me what type of activities they previously participated in and what they liked about the activities to help me create individualized physical activity plans that were more likely to be successful. For example, if a new member was a rower in college, he or she might enjoy our new state-of-the-art rowing machine.

If a new member liked dance, he or she might like our dance classes. We encouraged new members to rediscover a type or form of physical activity they enjoyed doing in their past and/or reconnect with an old friend they used to play tennis with or swim with. It was fun to see many new members take a walk down memory lane, recalling how active they once were. Many who were very active in their younger years would ask themselves aloud, "How did I let my health go and become so inactive!" A former college football player, for example, was "enlightened" by the fact that he was now totally inactive. The simple question of asking what he did in the past motivated him to get moving again. At the same time, he understood he was not 20 years of age anymore and needed to have a physical activity plan that would "match" his current level of fitness.

An Activity History helps you rediscover your favorite types of physical activity. When you complete your Activity History, try to rediscover or discover a type of physical activity that you may want to reincorporate into your life on a regular basis.

Perhaps an activity can trigger Dramatic Relief for you (Chapter 2). For example, on my 40th birthday, my beloved father gave me the most endearing gift: a hula hoop. My father recalled how I used to love to hula hoop when I was younger. This gift aroused a well of positive emotions inside of me, reminding me of happy, carefree, sunny summer days, hula hooping in my back yard with a smile! As an adult, I then resumed hula hooping in my own yard as one of my summer Return to Recess activities.

Journal Activity

Are there activities that trigger positive emotions in you? Take your time to think, and write down a few ideas in your journal. If not, completing an Activity History will help you Return to Recess! Follow this three-step process:

Step 1: Complete Your Activity History

1. What fun activities did you enjoy as a child that you can pick up again or continue?
2. What fun activities as a teenager and young adult could you pick up again or continue?
3. What fun activities have you always wanted to try?
4. What activities are you interested in doing to Return to Recess?

Step 2: Make a to-do list of two to four things to help you achieve your Return to Recess and physical activity goals

1.
2.
3.
4.

Step 3: Sign a "Return to Recess" Commitment Contract and stick to it!

Making a Commitment Contract entails believing in your ability to change, and acting on that belief by making a commitment to altering your behavior. Here, you are using Self-Liberation by committing to your behavior change goals (Chapter 2).

Your "Return to Recess" Commitment Contract:

> *I commit to Return to Recess at least three times per week, between (insert hours or time), for at least 10 minutes per day starting (insert date). I will (list activities) or participate in any other fun physical activity.*
>
> *Signed:*

Let's look at a sample Activity History I completed to get an idea of how to fill one out.

Step 1: Complete an Activity History

1. What fun activities did you enjoy as a child that you can pick up again or continue?

    - Hula hooping.
    - Bike riding.

2. What fun activities as a teenager and young adult could you pick up again or continue?

    - Figure skating.
    - Dance exercising.
    - Weight training.

3. What fun activities have you always wanted to try?

    - Mini trampolining.
    - Paddle boarding.

4. What activities are you interested in doing to Return to Recess?

    - Hula hooping.
    - Mini trampolining.
    - Dance exercising breaks.
    - Boxing.

Step 2: Make a to-do list of two to four things that help you achieve your Return to Recess goals

- ↝ Buy a freestanding boxing bag.
- ↝ Put my hula hoop on the front porch where I can see it every day.
- ↝ Dust off and test my mini trampoline.
- ↝ Gather my favorite music together for my dance breaks.

Step 3: Sign a "Return to Recess" Commitment Contract and stick to it!

I commit to Return to Recess at least three times per week, between 2 a.m. and 4 p.m., for at least 10 minutes per day starting January 5, 2014. I will do my hula hooping, use my mini trampoline, take a dance break, or participate in any other fun physical activity.

Signed: Annie

Self-Expectations

Curiously enough, resurrecting your past activities, particularly if you were at a competitive athletic level, can result in shying away from those activities that you once excelled at and loved. Beau, a pharmaceutical executive, was a varsity rower at a prestigious college in the northeast. As you know, being a varsity collegiate level athlete requires a high degree of athletic and mental strength and ability. Now 40-something, Beau continues to work out regularly at a health club. We were discussing this book, and I began asking him, as a former rower and athlete, to tell me about his current physical activity routine. He shared with me his routine, and a curious observation was uncovered: For all these years, Beau had always ignored and purposely stayed away from the rowing machine at the health club. Recently, one of the new trainers at the health club learned that Beau was a varsity rower in college and encouraged him to give it a try. Beau was reluctant. He was at such a high level of performance in college, he felt that rowing was part of his past, something to be left behind. As a former competitive figure skater, I understood. I had a lot of difficulty returning to skating recreationally, although I really enjoy skating.

Accepting the reality that you are not at the same performance level that you once were at a different time and place in your life, now with other priorities, can be difficult. I needed to shift my self-expectation from being a high-level, competitive figure skater to a recreational skater. This was not easy. I needed to accept this fact and put my ego aside, as it played a role in my negative feelings about myself. I needed to focus on the enjoyment of the activity, skating, not about my previous level of performance in my younger years. Beau's shared a similar experience. Once he accepted this was a different time, and had different expectations of himself, he got on that rower. Beau immediately and instinctively had the rowing form of that collegiate athlete, and he began to feel good about resurrecting his past activity.

If you can gain acceptance of who and where you are right now in time, perhaps a bit older, with more of life's demands, and let go of the competitiveness that may have once accompanied a previous activity of yours, you may reconnect with the activity and find yourself enjoying it even more! You can re-engage because of your pure love and enjoyment of the activity without concern for competiveness. To this day, Beau uses and enjoys the rowing machine regularly and "gets lost" in the steady motion of the activity that captivated him as a young man with a tight-knit group of team members. By resurrecting one of your favorite activities, competitive or not, you may create fond memories that can transcend decades.

Making the Time for Return to Recess

The number-one barrier to the commitment of engaging in a healthy lifestyle that I hear from individuals, health coaches, and health club trainers is lack of time. Return to Recess is designed to make you want to find the time, because it's fun and it is easier to find short bouts of time for physical activity. Think back on everything you have done this week. Have you ever spent time with someone or spent time doing something like watching television because it was fun or you enjoyed it? That is the goal of Return to Recess. You do it because you *want* to—because it's *fun* for *you*!

Tips for Keeping your Commitment Contract

- ↝ Identify your best time for recess. Pick a time that works well with your schedule or rearrange your schedule to accommodate it and stick to it. What time works best for you? Midafternoon works well for me. It allows me to put in a full morning of work and break for lunch, and, just before the afternoon slump, I Return to Recess and play for a short time while having fun!

- Schedule your recess time. Schedule and block out the best time(s) in your iPhone or calendar. Set an alarm or post visual reminders in multiple places.

- Create your favorite music playlist. Listen to it when you Return to Recess. This will help you look forward to that time.

- Identify friends, family members, or colleagues to join you on recess. Remember recess periods when you couldn't wait to play and see your friends? Are there friends, family members, or family pets that you can enjoy your recess activities with? Having recess with others also strengthens your Helping Relationships, a Process of Change (chapters 2 and 4). What friends, family members, and pets can you Return to Recess with? Can you shoot hoops or play catch with your child (young *or* adult!) or spouse? Can you go for a quick walk with a colleague? Can you walk or play ball with your dog for 10 minutes outside?

- Pick a daily verbal cue for recess. Pick and say aloud a verbal cue at your designated Return to Recess time (research related to verbal cues is presented in Chapter 5). Some examples include "It's MY TIME!" or "The work can wait, let's walk!" Other examples include "It's FUN time!" or "Yay, it's time to PLAY!" What are your verbal cues?

Sample Activities for Returning to Recess

Some of these activities may be done during recess or may take longer and be considered for regular physical activity routines if you are in the *action* stage of change:

- Walking
- Trampolining
- Jump roping

- Playing Frisbee
- Swimming
- Playing tennis
- Rollerblading
- Biking
- Skiing (downhill or cross county)
- Snowshoeing
- Paddle boarding
- Playing catch
- Playing basketball or shooting hoops
- Going to the playground with your children, using swings
- Playing horseshoes
- Playing volleyball
- Bowling
- Playing badminton
- Playing bocce ball

What can you add to this list?

Ready for Action?

If you are preparing for or ready to take action on a more formal physical activity program, use your Activity History to begin to explore physical activity options that appeal to you. You could also sample activities "buffet style," by choosing from a variety of options to find the right activities for you that you will want to continue doing long-term.

Buffet-Style Matchmaking

When new members came into my health club, I encouraged them to sample each piece of physical activity equipment for five minutes throughout the course of a week, and try as many classes, with as many different instructors, as possible. This "buffet-style" approach allowed members to get a "taste" of all physical activity options available to them to find their physical activity "match" or type of physical activity that they really liked, and found enjoyable and fun! Finding your perfect "match" related to *any* type of positive behavior options may take some time.

Like dating, you may have to "date" and meet a variety of physical activity options for some time before you find your match. If you don't find it immediately, keep looking to meet alternatives. After working with hundreds of individuals throughout the years, I couldn't say how many times I have heard "I tried exercising at a gym, but I hated it" or "I tried yoga (or other physical activity class) and didn't enjoy it." The key is not to get discouraged and stop, as each gym, health club, or fitness facility is different, each class and instructor is different, and each type of physical activity equipment (indoors or out) is different. There is no "one size fits all" when it comes to physical activity options and I have sadly seen too many people give up too soon. Keep trying options, and give yourself time to find your physical activity match(es). Some of my health club members loved the treadmill, whereas others despised it. Some even said they felt like they were on a hamster wheel when using the treadmill, going nowhere, and really wanted to walk or run outdoors. Others loved the steady cadence of the treadmill. So, when you are ready for *action* and a more regular physical activity routine than Return to Recess, take adequate time for you to sample a variety of options to find your perfect match for both the type of physical activity as well as type of equipment (if equipment is needed). What are some physical activity options that you could try?

Your "Gym Uniform"

I can still see my junior high school gym uniform, the navy blue, pinstriped polyester top and gym shorts in a clear plastic bag. In my high school days, we were required to change into our gym uniforms before we went to gym class. Although I despised that uniform, it was effective at switching my mindset from the classroom setting to physical activity time. Although it was comfortable and easy to exercise in, it was not very fashionable. Who picked out those gym uniforms, anyway? But seriously, when you are ready for more formal or regular physical activity, it is a good idea to get and use a "gym uniform." Besides putting you in an *action* frame of mind, your "uniform" or dedicated workout clothes can psych you up for a better workout. A good workout outfit will allow for improved flexibility, freedom of movement, and comfort with not a lot of material to slow you down. It must not be baggy. I recommend that your "gym uniform" be at least somewhat flattering to help make you feel good about yourself while working out. Often, members came into my health club wearing baggy, "frumpy" sweats. If a large majority of these same members were asked how they felt in their workout clothes, they was reply "not very good." However, once many of these members invested in fashionable and comfortable clothing that were more form-fitting and flattering, even if they were overweight, they said they felt and performed much better! They were much happier during and after their workouts!

One does not need to spend a fortune on their "gym uniform." Many discount and second-hand stores have very affordable and attractive options. There are many sales on the Internet as well. The key is to first try on several different styles and brands to ensure you feel comfortable in them and they flatter you. The way you feel about yourself while you work out will really affect your performance and put you in the right frame of mind. Remember: "Change Your Mind, Change Your Health!"

Your Workout "Experience"

Change Your Environment: Create a Sensory Experience

Club Med provides an "experience" that combines sports and relaxation, a healthy combination that can enhance a workout experience. Creating an environment at home, or finding a health club that supports an experience similar to Club Med's may enhance your physical activity adherence. The goal is to motivate you to *want* to be physically active, as opposed to feeling like you *have* to be physically active. Enhance your environment to support your change. In addition, make your workout a sensory experience. Creating an environment that appeals to your senses can create a positive distraction and make your experience more enjoyable. Perhaps you just need a "mental" Return to Recess day by engaging in a sensory activity to reduce your stress and improve your mood. Engaging your senses may provide a therapeutic affect to prepare you for activity later or to restore your energy so you may Return to Recess the next day.

Engage Your Senses!

Sense is defined by Merriam-Webster as one of the five natural powers (touch, taste, smell, sight, and hearing) through which you receive information about the world around you. Your senses have a powerful affect on your physical and emotional being. Keep in mind that you can activate your senses in a positive way to enhance your behavior change. Discover ways to engage your senses to create a fun, positive environment and experience to help you Return to Recess, physically *or* mentally!

Tips for Engaging Your Senses

Hearing

Whether you wish to change your sedentary lifestyle, poor eating habits, smoking, stress, or any other problem behavior, music can provide a relaxing, motivating experience. Research has shown that listening to music before an activity can activate arousal or increased motivation to change. So, if you don't feel like Returning to Recess when you get home, put on your favorite CD or playlist to motivate you. Research has shown that music produces an "arousal" effect and motivates us to move; it also reduces our perception of effort and significantly increases our endurance during exercise (Karageorghis and Priest, 2012). In addition, the right music can help relieve your stress and positively influence your mood when needed.

Small water gardens with gentle waterfall sounds or ambient noise can provide a relaxation response, helping you reduce stress and get ready to Return to Recess. Managing your stress levels will also help you have more energy for physical activity and for *fun*!

Sight

Motivational posters or other visual prompts such as pictures of your favorite places, or pictures of you participating in activities alone or with family members or friends, can create an environment conducive to physical activity.

Use notes or sticky notes to remind you of your scheduled Return to Recess time. Use warm light or sunlight to help sooth you.

Touch

Keep your favorite lotions handy in your office, car, or purse to apply or massage on dry skin throughout the day. Scented lotions will also engage your sense of smell.

Pet your cat or dog. Take a hot bath or shower. Hot water on your skin provides an immediate relaxation response. Wrap yourself up in a warm blanket or in a favorite, cozy robe on a cold day.

Smell

Use scented candles, lotions, incense, or air fresheners. Sip hot, flavored, scented teas or cider. Cook a healthy, flavorful meal and savor the scents.

Taste

Taste is a powerful sense that is critical to enjoying your food. If you are looking to change your dietary habits, experiment with different healthy recipes with different flavors and spices. One barrier to healthy eating is the misperception that healthy foods are not tasty.

Sip a cup of your favorite flavor of tea to engage your senses of taste *and* smell. Also, touching a warm cup or mug makes tea time even more comforting on a chilly day!

Multisensory

Many of the tips listed here can engage multiple senses. The more the better, so enjoy!

Change your scenery. Go outdoors, away from mental distractions, and immerse yourself in pleasant sights or views, the brush of fresh air on your skin, the warmth of the sun upon your face. "Take time to smell the roses."

Return to Recess is about taking a break from your workday or your everyday routine to improve or maintain your mental *and* physical well-being. Physically active recess is ideal, but some days we may just need a mental recess. Either is okay. In later chapters, I will discuss how we move to *action* and commit to regular and more moderate and vigorous activity needed to get results. The goal of Return to Recess is to have fun and engage in activities that make you move, happy, and smile! It is that simple!

Key Points

- Return to Recess can be enjoyed by all, no matter what your Stage of Change!
- Sample a variety of activities to find the right "match."
- Enjoyment and satisfaction lead to improved adherence to any chosen activity.
- Activate your environment to create an engaging experience.
- Engage all your senses.

Action Items

- Complete your Activity History to rediscover or discover fun activities.
- Return to Recess at least three days per week.
- Complete your Commitment Contract.

4

Building Confidence Through Mastery

Insider Secret #4:
Improve Confidence to Change:
The Self-Efficacy Theory

Alex, an FBI agent who joined my health club, asked me to work with her one-on-one on a weight loss program. Alex represented herself as a confident woman. She was a solid, large-framed, physically fit woman, but wanted to lose 20 pounds. Her job evolved to include more administrative responsibilities as she came off "field duty" the prior year. As a result of these increased responsibilities and job promotion, Alex was less active, spending longer sedentary hours at her desk, and gained weight. Alex tried on many occasions to lose weight but was not successful. She stated that she didn't have the confidence that she needed for successful weight loss without personal coaching. I thought to myself, *Alex is an FBI agent. Why does she need MY help? How could Alex NOT be confident?* FBI agents are some of the most confident and self-disciplined individuals. I was totally perplexed!

Through my own journey and the journeys of those I worked with and continue to work with, I learned about the difference between self-esteem and self-efficacy. Self-esteem is related to an individual's perception of his or her overall self-worth. Self-efficacy, on the other hand, is the confidence in one's ability to accomplish specific tasks. They are two very different things. So, although Alex was a very confident individual with high self-esteem, her self-efficacy in achieving and maintaining weight loss was low. Self-efficacy is situational. It is a measure of the belief in one's own ability to complete *certain tasks* and to achieve *certain goals* under *certain circumstances*. If you are aware of what you believe about your own ability to change a certain behavior, or to accomplish certain tasks needed to accomplish your goals you can consciously take control of the outcome. You can create a workable blueprint to increase your own self-efficacy by creating manageable goals, and drawing on other sources that will lead to a greater sense of self-confidence to accomplish them.

The outcome of self-efficacy is based on your personal beliefs related to your action(s). These beliefs will determine what course(s) of action you may or may not pursue, such as whether or not to lose weight. Other factors that affect your action or inaction include how much effort you will need to exert to achieve your goal (for example, weight loss, quit smoking), how long you will have to persevere when facing barriers, previous failures or other future obstacles, your resilience in the face of adversity, the positivity or negativity of your thinking or thoughts, how much stress and depression you experience as you pursue your goals, and your belief in the level of success and/or accomplishments you will achieve along the way. All these influences play a role in achieving and sustaining a high degree of self-efficacy for permanent behavior change.

This chapter introduces Bandura's self-efficacy theory of behavior change (1997), another construct or component of the Transtheoretical Model (TTM). I applied this theory extensively to change my own health behaviors, and I have taught hundreds of individuals and groups throughout my career how to apply it as well. I have been privileged to witness many individuals leverage this theory to change their health by changing their minds. Research has repeatedly shown that if you believe you have the confidence to perform a task, your chance of success is greater. This chapter will explain the Four Sources of Self-Efficacy and how to draw on these sources, just as successful sports and life coaches use them, to help you build and sustain the confidence needed to achieve your goals (Warner, Schüz, Knittle, Zielgelmann, and Wurm, 2011). The information you gain through the Sources of Self-Efficacy is pertinent to judging your capabilities to perform and successfully change a health behavior. As you process information on these sources, and think about and reflect on their relative importance, you may improve your confidence or self-efficacy. Pure knowledge, skills, tools, and/or support will not produce successful results if we lack the self-assurance to use them. We need confidence in our abilities to utilize or apply the resources we have to succeed. Knowing does not equate to doing!

The Four Sources of Self-Efficacy

The Four Sources of Self-Efficacy include the following and are described following:

- Mastery Experience.
- Vicarious Experience or Observational Learning.
- Verbal Persuasion.
- Physiological and Emotional Cues and Responses.

These sources have been shown through decades of research to improve one's confidence to achieve specific tasks or goals. As you strive to change a health behavior, turn to these sources for the *power* to increase your confidence (Bandura, 1997).

Mastery Experience

Jenny tried every weight-loss diet imaginable on her own before working with her new health coach, Tom. She lost weight on many of these diets, only to regain the weight, and sometimes more, upon returning to her normal lifestyle. This is a common story. Jenny would always be optimistic when starting a new weight-loss program, but was unaware of how past "failures" negatively influenced her self-efficacy. She consistently started out well, but underneath she believed "this time would not be any different." Tom understood how important it was for Jenny to be aware of how her past experiences influenced her current self-beliefs so he did not immediately design a weight-loss program with her. Instead, Tom spent time discussing Jenny's past experiences to help Jenny "enlighten" herself as to how she truly felt about herself, and her failed efforts *and* successes, before they were ready to move ahead. Together, they created a blueprint for a weight-loss program based on *small* and *attainable* achievements, ultimately increasing Jenny's self-efficacy through mastery experience for weight-loss and weight loss maintenance.

Although Jenny still struggled at times, she was able to feel more in control by accepting that failed weight-loss attempts were in the past and were actually valuable experiences that could facilitate or help lead to future success. Jenny found herself so focused on past failures she had forgotten her past successes! As she began succeeding at achieving smaller and more realistic milestones that she set with Tom, she was ready to move on to more structured and challenging nutrition and physical activity goals. Jenny learned to focus on past and current successes, and this time spent more time in *preparation*. Jenny also mentally prepared herself for increased self-efficacy and positive and sustained health behavior change.

Mastery Experience is our personal experience with success or failure. Most of us are aware of the common recommendation to break larger goals or tasks into smaller, more achievable goals for success. This approach is designed to result in increased self-efficacy and positive Mastery Experience through a single success or repeated successes, no matter how small or large we perceive them to be. What a great feeling! Bandura's research found that Mastery Experience is the most powerful source of self-efficacy. The mastering of a task provides "the most authentic confidence of whether one can muster up whatever it takes to succeed" (Bandura, 1997, p. 80). In order to achieve and sustain positive health behavior change, we must garner experience in overcoming obstacles. When we face challenges related to a problem behavior that we are actively seeking to change, and successfully conquer them over time, we develop a resilient, behavior-specific sense of mastery and self-efficacy.

Using Mastery Experience to Improve Self-Efficacy

- ↝ Break down your ultimate goal into smaller steps.
- ↝ Recognize your small achievements as success.
- ↝ Focus and build on your past successes (as opposed to negatively focusing on past "failures").
- ↝ Reflect on positive outcomes and lessons learned from past perceived "failures."
- ↝ Strategize and plan for ways to overcome potential obstacles and barriers.

Journal Activity

Ask yourself the following questions:

- ❧ What are three successful accomplishments that I have made in the past?
- ❧ Thinking of these accomplishments, what are some common themes have helped me achieve my goal?
- ❧ How can I apply these common themes to my *current* health behavior change?

Tips for Creating a Past and Present List of Mastery Experiences

- ❧ Make a list of the personal health behavior changes you have mastered.
- ❧ As you prepare to change a current health behavior, remind yourself of those achievements.
- ❧ Think about how you can apply the successful components of your past achievements to your current goal.

Sample Past List of Mastery Experiences

- ❧ I lost and kept off 15 pounds.
- ❧ I was once able to stop smoking for two days.
- ❧ I kept to a routine of eight hours of sleep every night for three weeks.
- ❧ I adhered to my doctor's orders and took my medications regularly for more than two months.
- ❧ I did sit-ups every night for six months to tighten my abdominal muscles.
- ❧ I completed yoga exercises three times per week for a month.

Sample Present List of Mastery Experiences

Keep a daily list of your current accomplishments, as "small" as you think they may be.

- Returned to Recess for 10 minutes this afternoon.
- Ate a healthy breakfast.
- Drank six glasses of water.
- Walked my dog.
- Read a "success story."
- Subscribed to a credible health magazine.
- Did not consume any alcoholic beverages at this evening's dinner party.

Journal Activity

Ask yourself the following questions:

- What are some common themes that helped me achieve these tasks?
- How can I apply these common themes to my *current* health behavior change?
- What are some ways that I can break down my health behavior goal into smaller steps or milestones?

Vicarious Experience or Observational Learning

Early in my career, I worked as a trainer at the Newport Athletic Club in Middletown, Rhode Island. In 1983, the America's Cup race was hosted in Newport, Rhode Island. The America's Cup crews all trained at the Club, and different teams from all over the world were bused in each morning at about the same time. Italy, France, the United States, Australia, and other countries all worked out in the same room, creating a "Vicarious Experience" for crew members. Vicarious Experience is also known as Observational Learning. In simple terms, Observational Learning results in learning from and being motivated by observing the successes of others—most importantly, individuals we are similar to or can relate to (Bandura, 1997). Observational Learning can provide a greater incentive and result in increased self-efficacy and motivation for one to strive for his or her best. Often, people compare their own abilities to the abilities or attainments of others. When we watch people similar to us engage in a positive health behavior, we may say, "If they can do it, I can do it!"

When comparing your performance related to a particular health behavior to another person's, it is important to be realistic. Observational Learning can be contraindicated if we compare ourselves to those whose abilities and behaviors are "out of our league." For example, if we are just beginning a physical activity program and compare ourselves to someone 30 years younger than us and with optimal physical conditioning or fitness, we can easily get discouraged. However, for optimal self-efficacy and to motivate us to achieve our goals, it is not only important for us to challenge ourselves with the benchmarks of others practicing the same health behaviors and with a similar level of experience, but also to seek to observe and learn from those at a higher Stage of Change. Certainly in sports and in other life experiences, challenging and surpassing a comparable competitor may raise self-efficacy, but being consistently outperformed may lower it.

As discussed in Chapter 1, I gained weight from an unhealthy lifestyle while working as a consultant in the health and wellness field! My colleague Linda and I both had excessive travel demands to frequently meet with clients nationwide, lack of consistent access to healthy foods, and poor sleep schedules due to the nature of our jobs. Yet, Linda had been consulting for 10 years longer than I and was able to maintain a healthy lifestyle, in spite all of the demands of the job. When Linda arrived at hotels, she always had a soft cooler that contained fresh fruit, nuts, and other healthy snacks. On trips to meet our current and potential clients, I observed how Linda ate her own healthy snacks, fit morning walks into her schedule before our client meetings, and planned healthy dinner choices by reviewing the menu prior to a business dinner with a client. I felt if Linda could do it, I could do it as well! Through Observational Learning, Linda helped improve my self-efficacy by showing me how I could make healthy choices in the midst of numerous barriers. Thank you, Linda!

When I observed Linda, I was in *preparation* to make healthier choices. I just needed the self-efficacy to successfully act on them. I had to be open to observing Linda's health behaviors and able to identify with Linda and her work situation in order to be able to make similar healthy lifestyle choices. When striving for health behavior change, observe the pertinent health behaviors of others that possess similar skills or are in similar situations as you. Observe those who are succeeding at behavior change and explore ways for you to model their behaviors.

Use Observational Learning to Accomplish Your Goals

- ❧ Join a gym, exercise class, or group to motivate you to work harder.
- ❧ Observe the healthy behaviors of others to provide you with opportunities to improve your self-efficacy.
- ❧ Watch videos or read testimonials about people like you, working toward achieving the same goal, and in a similar situation or facing the same barriers as you.
- ❧ Follow and contribute to relevant YouTube and/or Twitter users or other social networking sites specific to your goal (for example, SparkPeople.com, WeightWatchers.com).
- ❧ Subscribe to credible health magazines or online resources and read the testimonials about the successes of others like you.

Journal Activity

Ask yourself the following questions:

- ❧ Is there someone I know who has accomplished or is accomplishing the goals I wish to achieve? Can I observe how they are achieving their goals?
- ❧ Where am I able to observe and model the behaviors of others like me (for example, gym, yoga class, work)?

Verbal Persuasion

Once Tom, the Rhode Island state employee discussed in Chapter 2, successfully walked one corridor in the State House consistently without getting winded, he achieved a sense of mastery over walking. Even though Tom didn't complete the walking route in its entirety, he broke down the task and completed the first goal of one corridor. He then started routinely walking with several colleagues and was able to expand his walk to the second corridor. In just a few weeks, Tom mastered both corridors and achieved his ultimate goal of walking the entire first floor of the State House. By breaking down the goal into smaller and very doable tasks, Tom improved his self-efficacy through accumulating Mastery Experience. If Tom had attempted to do too much too soon and was unsuccessful, he would have compromised his sense of mastery as well as self-efficacy.

Another important factor that helped improve Tom's self-efficacy was the "Verbal Persuasion" he received throughout the program. From the very beginning, Sue, the Wellness Champion for the State House, walked side by side with Tom and accompanied him at his own pace. Sue encouraged Tom by telling him he could successfully accomplish his goal of becoming more physically active. As time progressed and Tom began walking with other colleagues, he received encouragement in the form of Verbal Persuasion from them as well. Eventually, Tom inspired and walked with *others* who came to start the program at the same level of self-efficacy that Tom originally had. Newcomers to the program, in turn, offered Tom even *more* support, continually increasing their *and* Tom's self-efficacy for daily walking. As a result of participating in the State House walk for six months or so, Tom was able to join his colleagues on a much anticipated bus trip to New York City to see a Broadway play—a reward that, in Tom's words shared with Sue, transformed his life.

Journal Activity

Make a list of people to include family, friends, colleagues, neighbors, or anyone that you can call on to support you and provide Verbal Persuasion during your journey of behavior change. Try to think of everyone, even someone you may have shared a similar goal with in the past. Next to their names, list what they may be able to help you with. If your goal is physical fitness, ask friends who are physically active on a regularly basis. Ask them to share their routine, what works for them, and any ideas on how they may be able to support you to get started on your journey. Through your Helping Relationships (Chapter 2), share your current Stage of Change for the behavior that you are seeking support for, your short- and long-term "mastery" goals, and ask for assistance.

Don't be afraid to ask for help! Social support works the best when the people who are supporting you understand what and how much support you need, as well as what you don't need. I have asked friends of mine that consistently practice healthy eating behaviors for their support with healthy recipe selections and other ideas for positive dietary changes, but I also explained my wishes to not be judged for my desire to not significantly limit my food choices.

Physiological and Emotional Cues and Responses

As a research associate at the University of Rhode Island from 1998 to 2005, one of the projects I worked on was to study the relationship between physical activity and fall prevention among inpatient psychiatric patients. As you might imagine, the use of health behavior change techniques to motivate patients to be physically active was a critical component of this work. One of my patients, Arthur, was a former construction worker who was accustomed to being physically active. Arthur was a quiet, soft-spoken man with soft blue eyes. His skin appeared rough and weathered from years of outdoor labor. Because of his previous career requiring years of physical labor, I assumed Arthur would be motivated to be physically active with his peers. I was wrong. Arthur reluctantly came to the onsite physical activity classes and usually left after the first five minutes to return to sitting and watching television.

After one of the classes ended, I went to sit with Arthur, asked him what he was watching on television, and asked why he left the group. Arthur simply starred at the television and shrugged his shoulders. I sat for a few minutes longer trying to engage Arthur in small talk. Being unsuccessful, I told Arthur the class would be offered again next week and, as always, invited him to join us. For the next three to four weeks Arthur chose not to participate in any of the physical activity classes and, each week after class, I attempted to engage Arthur in a small conversation about his resistance to participating.

After the fourth week, Arthur revealed that he did not like the way he felt in the physical activity classes. He became anxious when he felt his heart rate increasing. Knowing that Arthur suffered from panic attacks, I asked him if the feelings he experienced during class were similar. Arthur agreed. Arthur experienced the same physiological responses to physical activity as he did to panic attacks. On top of that, Arthur shared that his doctors would medicate him during a panic attack, which made him feel even worse about himself. With Arthur's willingness to open up about his feelings, I immediately understood! The physiological response Arthur was experiencing during physical activity was preventing him from participating, lowering his self-efficacy.

After a month or so of getting to know Arthur better and developing a mutually trusting relationship, I asked him to come back to the physical activity classes. I informed him that I would change his routine to make it more comfortable for him and told him he could stop at any time. My goal was to change Arthur's *perception* of the physiological responses preventing him from being physically active, *not* to suppress or eliminate the responses altogether. Arthur began to start the physical activity classes at a lower intensity, increasing his Mastery Experience. His Mastery Experience also helped him learn that his heart was working to make him healthier, exercise was doing him good, and he was not having a panic attack. After class, I used Verbal Persuasion to assure Arthur that the physiological feelings of a moderately increased heart rate during physical activity were actually positive. In addition, by participating in the physical activity classes, Arthur provided an opportunity for Observational Learning by other participating residents facing similar challenges. Throughout the course of a just a few weeks, I observed an increase in Arthur's emotional as well as physiological self-efficacy to be physically active. This experience at this residential treatment facility was very valuable to me, and working with the residents was one of the most rewarding projects in my career. Prior, I didn't realize the past and current trauma individuals with psychiatric illness live with and/or relive every day. I learned a great deal from witnessing this transformation within Arthur after he received the support and encouragement that he needed. Even a barrier such as a mental or psychiatric illness may be overcome to achieve positive health behavior change with the proper social and environmental supports.

Several members of my health club also struggled with their perception of their physiological responses to being physically active. If a new member didn't return to the club after a week of joining, I, or one of my staff, would try reach out to him or her. Sometimes, non-returning new members would explain that they were really sore after their first workout, or they "pushed themselves too hard" and could not think of immediately returning. Some new members felt they were so out of shape it was hopeless, and questioned whether they could or even wanted to continue. Even with resistance, my staff and I tried to encourage new members to start out slow (to gain Mastery Experience), and to have a safe, effective, and pleasant experience. We explained that individuals embarking on a physical activity program (or any other type of new health behavior program) needed to give their body a chance to adapt to the changes or new experiences.

Over a consistent amount of time with a new physical activity program, volume and intensity can be increased at a reasonable, safe, and effective pace. Some individuals may get "caught up in the moment" and start to prematurely increase the level or intensity of their workouts. When our endorphins kick in and we feel strong, it may be easy to forget to stay at the recommended level of frequency, intensity, and duration. This may be especially true when we expect fast results (for example, rapid weight loss). Unfortunately, this untamed motivation, without adequate recovery time, may have the opposite effect of extended muscle soreness and stiffness, demoralization, decreased self-efficacy, and the "crash and burn" feeling of defeat. But again, it's not the physical response that matters, but how we interpret these responses that affects our self-efficacy. When it comes to self-efficacy, our perceptions of our emotional responses are just as important as our perceptions of our physiological responses.

Since the day I was baptized Anna Maria Angelina Ludovici, my close Italian and Portuguese family has always celebrated life's special events, including every Sunday in my youth, with a feast! Our dining room table was like an altar; the place where we gathered to celebrate with a large variety of wonderful, beautifully prepared, and calorie-rich Italian foods. I learned, at a very early age, to *love* food! Considering my family background, and genes, maintaining a healthy lifestyle and body weight has always been a personal as well as professional concern of mine. As a result of my love for food, I try to avoid buffets. But when I do enter one, especially an all-you-can-eat buffet, I can feel myself becoming stressed and nervous. In addition to this emotional response,

I sometimes even experience a physiological response and can actually feel my heart beat faster. As I am writing this chapter, I am on a much-needed four-day getaway rock and roll cruise (more on that later). And, of course, cruises are known for their all-you-can-eat buffets!

Although my self-efficacy regarding the ability to not have a strong physiological response to buffets has improved substantially over time, as well as my Mastery Experience, I still would rather not eat at them because I have not yet *fully* mastered my emotional responses of stress and anxiety to the extent where I feel totally comfortable partaking in them. Because of the difficulty of avoiding buffets on a cruise, I am acknowledging my emotions while reassuring myself that I can and will control my portion sizes as well as selection of healthy food choices. This self-reassurance and self-verbal persuasion help me change my perception of these emotions and increase my self-efficacy to eat healthy at buffets. Because self-efficacy can vary or fluctuate with situations and environments, it is important that we acknowledge both our physiological and emotional cues to develop individualized strategies that work for us. In any uncomfortable situation, in addition to acknowledging my emotional state in a nonjudgmental way, I take some deep, relaxing breaths and also try to assess if my "automatic thoughts" or mental responses are realistic (Chapter 5), then execute my predetermined "game plan" for overcoming any potential barriers (Chapter 6).

As the director of the governor of Rhode Island's wellness initiative, *Get Fit Rhode Island!*, I frequently observed the governor's "advance person" arrive at a location an hour or so before the governor was scheduled to visit. This individual would ensure that every detail related to the governor, from his personal safety to his personal preferences, was accommodated. The reality is that most of us have to be our own "advance person" and prepare in advance, at least mentally, to make the safest and healthiest choices for ourselves. To overcome my barrier of buffets, I become my own advance person by viewing all of the possible choices *before* picking up a plate and decide on my selections in advance. Knowing and deciding in advance what my choices are helps me control my portion sizes, make better selections, and reduce my negative response to emotional cues; this protects my self-efficacy in these situations.

Each of us may perceive our situational responses differently. The goal is not to suppress or eliminate our responses, but to acknowledge them, and redirect or "reprogram" our thoughts if they are hindering us. Even if I "change" how I interpret my physiological and emotional responses to buffets, my mood will affect my self-efficacy. Our state of mood plays a critical role in how we judge our past, current, and future situations. If I am in a bad mood, I am more likely to be less "efficacious" about my abilities to control my portions and make healthy selections at a buffet. In this case, it would be best to avoid a buffet altogether until my mood improves, and use Stimulus Control, the Process of Change that helps us control situations and other causes that trigger a problem behavior (Chapter 2).

When we judge our capabilities to accomplish specific tasks, we partially rely on how we react to our body's responses, both physically and emotionally. In other words, our physiological and emotional responses can dictate our self-efficacy to accomplish certain things (Bandura, 1997). So, if we feel winded, fatigued, pain, stressed, or depressed, or experience other physical or emotional responses engaging in any healthy behavior change, our self-efficacy will be reduced *if* we interpret these responses negatively. How we *interpret* physiological and emotional responses is crucial to our success.

Journal Activity

Ask yourself:

- What physiological and or emotional responses do I observe while engaging in a new health behavior or changing a health behavior?
- How do I interpret these positive or negative responses?
- If I experience negative physiological or emotional responses, how can I "reframe" or positively interpret them to improve my self-efficacy?

The extent to which you can improve your experiences, performance, and self-efficacy through the Sources of Self-Efficacy depend on factors such as the following:

- ❧ Your preconceptions of your abilities.
- ❧ Your perceived level of difficulty of or amount of effort required for changing or engaging in a behavior.
- ❧ The amount of external help or social support you receive.
- ❧ Situational circumstances.
- ❧ Your interpretation of successes and "failures."

We must be *self-aware to self-change*. We must be aware of how we are judging ourselves, how we are complimenting ourselves, how much effort we are expending, and the resources and opportunities available to us. We are able to draw on the Sources of Self-Efficacy to change our health behaviors for good!

Self-Efficacy Activity

Complete the following confidence ruler to rate how confident you are in your ability to achieve your health behavior change goal. A number of situations listed can make it hard to stick to behavior change goals. On a scale of 0 to 100, please rate your confidence or self-efficacy in each of the blanks regarding how certain you are that you can get yourself to continue to practice your new or positive health behavior(s) on a regular basis during each of these situations (Pajares and Urdan, 2006).

Rate your degree of confidence by recording a number from 0 to 100 using the scale given below, with 0 being least efficacious and 100 being the most:

0   10   20   30   40   50   60   70   80   90   100

Cannot do at all   **Moderately can do**   **Highly certain can do**

_____When I am feeling tired

_____When I am feeling under pressure from work

_____During bad weather

_____After recovering from an injury that caused me to stop exercising

_____During or after experiencing personal problems

_____When I am feeling depressed

_____When I am feeling anxious

_____After recovering from an illness that caused me to stop exercising

_____When I feel physical discomfort when I exercise

_____After a vacation

_____When I have too much work to do at home

_____When visitors are present

_____When there are other interesting things to do

_____If I don't reach my exercise goals

_____Without the support from my family or friends

_____During a vacation

_____When I have other time commitments

_____After experiencing family problems

Rate your confidence regularly and use the sources of self-efficacy to improve your numbers.

Remember: Self-efficacy is task- and situation-specific, so you may want to complete the self-efficacy activity for all of the behaviors you wish to improve and in a variety of situations. For example, you may score a 90 in your confidence in the ability to exercise three times per week, but a 40 on your confidence in your ability to eat healthy on a daily basis. In addition, you may be faced with situations that make it difficult to stick to your health behavior change goal. Make a list of challenges that you may face on a regular basis when trying to achieve your health behavior change goal. The challenges on your list should vary in difficulty level, where some may be easier for you to overcome, and others may be more difficult. Next to each challenge, suggest solutions to overcome it or an alternative, positive health behavior that you could engage in. Possible solutions to the barriers listed are discussed in Chapter 6.

Key Points

- Self-efficacy regarding a specific health behavior is not the same as self-esteem.
- Self-efficacy is behavior- and situation-specific.

- The Four Sources of Self-Efficacy include Mastery Experience, Social Support, Vicarious Experience or Observational Learning, and the interpretation of Physiological and Emotional Cues.
- Mood influences self-efficacy.
- We must "be self-aware to self-change."

Action Items

- List your past and present Mastery Experiences.
- Improve your self-efficacy by applying the Four Sources of Self-Efficacy.
- Complete the Self-Efficacy Activity.

5

Change the Way You Think About It

Insider Secret #5:
Tips and Techniques to Change Mindsets

I can remember one gorgeous summer day when I tried to get my friend Jim, a crewmember for the America's Cup boat *Defender*, to play hooky from his daily workout and go to First Beach in Newport, Rhode Island, with other staff members from the health club. It was a perfect beach day. A light breeze was blowing and there wasn't a cloud in the sky. Jim was slightly tempted. Did he want a long indoor training session with a bunch of guys or an afternoon on one of the most beautiful beaches in New England? Jim chose the workout. At the time, I couldn't understand why. After all, he had been training all summer for these races. It was only one workout; why not miss it? However, after working with the crewmembers all summer, I learned to understand their dedication, and superior level of motivation and determination. I learned how they changed their thinking about decisions to eat healthy, not smoke, and avoid drinking alcohol to remain at peak physical and emotional well-being. Jim did not interpret foregoing to the beach with us as a sacrifice, but he did interpret taking the time off from training as one. He felt that if he gave up his workout, even just one, he would jeopardize his goals. Jim had positive thoughts about his workout. Like many athletes, Jim had the attitude that every day and every "play" count! To not compromise his workout goals, Jim stated he would hang out with us after his workout that day, and he did. Jim's example demonstrates we don't have to give up having fun or our social relationships to achieve our goals. It is possible, like Jim, to balance and do it all!

> *"What the mind of man can conceive and believe, it can achieve."*
> —Napoleon Hill

In this chapter, we will explore how our thinking affects our health behavior.

Let's begin by examining the power of our thoughts and how we can change our thoughts to change our emotions, our moods, and, ultimately, our health behavior. By heightening our awareness or mindfulness of our physical, mental, and emotional states, as well as our reactions to those states, we can empower ourselves to be better equipped to successfully navigate and manage situations and events. It is important to note that all of the techniques presented in this chapter may be effectively leveraged no matter what Stage of Change we are in.

Thoughts

> *"With the new day comes new strength and new thoughts."*
> —Eleanor Roosevelt

Identifying our thoughts and restructuring them is the basis of many effective techniques used in psychotherapeutic approaches such as Cognitive Behavioral Therapy (CBT). Researchers found that negative and/or distorted beliefs and thoughts affect emotions and behavior. There is a reciprocal relationship between them. Increased awareness of our thoughts that occur in response to situations, events, and interactions can help us improve our subsequent behavior. CBT has been demonstrated to be highly effective with health behavior change and the improvement of chronic illnesses (Hobbis and Sutton, 2005). Through my master's thesis research, "Examining the Addition of Cognitive Behavioral Strategies to a Standard Weight Loss Program," I found that weight-loss participants who used cognitive behavioral strategies and techniques significantly lost more weight throughout the course of the study, and sustained their weight loss longer, than those who participated in a standard weight-loss program.

More than five decades of research on CBT has shown that when people learn to process their thoughts in realistic, positive, and/or flexible ways, they experience optimal emotional, behavioral, and physical reactions to situations and events. These types of reactions, in turn, support positive behavior change. Negative, rigid, or limited thinking negatively influences our reactions to situations and events, impairing our ability to change. So, it is important for us to get a proper handle on our thoughts for positive and effective behavior change. By changing our thoughts, we can change our emotions and moods which, in turn, change our behavior. "Change your mind, change your health!"

Automatic Thoughts

"Automatic Thoughts" are thoughts that arise spontaneously. Sometimes our Automatic Thoughts "come out of the blue" and can be uncontrollable (Hobbis, et al., 2005). Therefore, these thoughts are termed "automatic," as they are not a result of deliberation or reasoning and are more reactionary (Beck, 2011). Often, we may not even be consciously aware of our Automatic Thoughts. Most of the time the thoughts are very brief, and we may be more aware of the emotions that arise from them than the thoughts themselves. Automatic Thoughts lead to reactions that affect our emotions and moods. It is not situations or events that determine how we feel, but how we interpret or analyze them. Therefore, becoming more mindful of our thoughts can assist us in interpretation of our thoughts, and in turn allows us to shift our way of thinking to not let distressing or negative thoughts jeopardize our behavior change actions and goals.

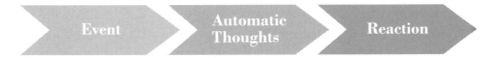

We may experience Automatic Thoughts when faced with a situation or event that influences our emotional and physiological reactions and, in turn, our behaviors. Automatic Thoughts drive our "knee-jerk reactions" to situations. The first step in controlling our Automatic Thoughts is to first identify what they are by increasing our awareness of them. It is also helpful to "distance" our thoughts and allow adequate time to evaluate them mindfully, as opposed to impulsively. Let's use the example where Jim from the America's Cup Crew was faced with the situation of being asked to skip his daily training routine.

1. A situation occurred: Jim was faced with a request to skip one day of his training to go to the beach or stay the course and complete it.

2. Automatic Thoughts occurred: Jim stated, "I want to work out, I need to work out, and I will hang out with you guys later." His immediate, knee-jerk reactions (Automatic Thoughts) were that he wanted to stay the course, that every workout counted, and deviating from his daily training routine was not an option. He wanted his team to win the Cup, and to Jim, each and every training routine was critical for success. Jim didn't feel deprived or "bummed." He was focused on his goal and self-determined.

3. A reaction to Automatic Thoughts occurred: Jim's positive thoughts and mood made him psyched for his workout. He was not disappointed or conflicted by his decision. Jim's resulting behavior, continuing his daily training routine, was maintained.

Jim's Automatic Thoughts could very well have been negative—for example, "I'm so tired of this demanding training routine," "I'm always missing out on everything because of this training," or "This sucks. I want to go to the beach!" Had Jim reacted impulsively, not mindfully, to coincide with his ultimate workout goal, these types of thoughts, along with his mood and emotions, may have ultimately resulted in a different outcome. There were other factors affecting how Jim reacted to this situation and how he controlled his thoughts and behavior. These factors and related theories and techniques that may be used to handle them will be introduced in Chapter 7.

Thought Records

The best way to become more aware of our Automatic Thoughts is to write them down. "Thought Records" help us track, evaluate, and redirect our thoughts when necessary. For the purposes of behavior change, Thought Records may be used to understand our Automatic Thoughts by enlightening us with a heightened awareness of our reactions to situations or events and to self-correct if necessary. Thought Records help us to better understand our thoughts and, ultimately, improve our moods, emotions, and behaviors. Thought Records may reveal that we may need to take another view of our automatic responses. They may also help us identify negative thought patterns. Pattern identification is particularly effective in maintaining positive behavior change. We cannot change what we are not aware of. Tracking and evaluating our reactions to situations or events help us better understand our behaviors so we can make appropriate adjustments to our automatic thought processes as needed. Thought Records help us change our health beliefs on a core level.

Journal Activity

Ask yourself, "What was going through my mind?" when:

- ↝ I felt stressed, anxious, or uncomfortable with a situation.
- ↝ I noticed physically distressing changes in my body.
- ↝ I felt inclined to react or behave in a negative way as opposed to a more rationale or positive way (Beck, 2011).

Restructure to Change!

A technique for changing our Automatic Thoughts is to restructure or reconstruct our reactions to situations. Thought restructuring is like the development of a rational rebuttal to Automatic Thoughts. By looking at a situation in a different way, we may rebuild or redirect our thoughts to support positive health behavior (Hope, Burns, Hayes, Herbert, and Warner, 2010). For example, upon entering an all-you-can-eat buffet, my previous Automatic Thought may have been something like, "Oh no, look at all the incredibly delicious food choices. I am going to overindulge!" However, by practicing mindfulness, and deep breathing, over time I have been able to cultivate more positive and rational thoughts in situations such as "I have been and I continue to be successful at maintaining my weight and healthy eating habits" or "You can do this Annie. Stop overgeneralizing and catastophizing!" By restructuring my thinking and drawing on other techniques described throughout this book, I have been able to successfully keep my portions under control, eat some of the more highly caloric foods I love in moderation, and "master the experience" of buffet-style eating. When in current situations that trigger Automatic Thoughts, I remind myself of how I have coped and adapted well in challenging situations that could have easily set me back or prevented me from achieving my goals. Although I am not always successful, my Mastery Experience and restructured thinking allow me to get right back on track more quickly. Positive self-affirmations such as "I can do this!" or "Annie, relax. You have done this many times!" have also been effective in restructuring my negative thinking to be more positive.

By consistently asking yourself the questions that follow, evaluating your Automatic Thoughts will become a natural process.

Evaluating Automatic Thoughts

The following questions listed may help you evaluate the validity of your Automatic Thoughts. Think of a recent difficult situation that made you question your self-efficacy in achieving your health goal. Think about your first Automatic Thought.

Journal Activity

Ask yourself:

- What is my evidence that my Automatic Thought is true? What is the evidence that it is false?
- Was there another way of looking at this situation? Can I think of a positive outcome from my experience?
- If there was a negative outcome, what was the worst thing that happened? How did I cope with the outcome? (Beck, 2011)

This may appear to be a difficult exercise at first. However, in time, and with objective practice, you will improve how you evaluate your Automatic Thoughts and how you constructively work through challenging situations and events by reframing or restructuring your Automatic Thought process.

In some cases, our Automatic Thoughts may be true. In these situations, it is important to focus on problem-solving. Sometimes it is difficult to see solutions to our problems or barriers ourselves, but we may leverage our resources for assistance. Resources may include our Helping Relationships or social supports (Chapter 2). They may include our family, friends, colleagues, neighbors, healthcare providers, employee assistance program, or social services or support groups available in the community and online. Self-help techniques for problem-solving and barrier removal are described in detail in Chapter 6. Once we identify our problems, we can work toward resolution. Problems or barriers do not equate to failure. They are simply "speed bumps" that may slow us down on our journey toward successful health behavior change!

In some cases, we need to be aware that our Automatic Thoughts may not be valid or may be distorted or exaggerated, so it's important to challenge our thoughts. When we evaluate situations and events, it is important to know if we are experiencing "Thinking Errors." Thinking Errors occur when we incorrectly interpret situations or events.

Some Automatic Thoughts may be considered dysfunctional because they can affect the interpretation of situations in a biased or exaggerated way (Hobbis, et al., 2005). Thinking Errors are erroneous conclusions or judgments that we may make about ourselves or events or situations. At one time or another, we may find ourselves judging ourselves or others irrationally, or jumping to erroneous conclusions. As we track and evaluate our thoughts, it is important to identify Thinking Errors as well as any patterns in type, frequency, and triggers of erroneous thinking. Once we are aware of our Thought Errors, triggers, and patterns, we may more successfully and expeditiously change a health behavior. There are ways to challenge these Thinking Errors and assess whether our Automatic Thoughts are indeed true, such as by putting the distortion on trial with probing questions. Types and examples of Thinking Errors and sample probing questions are listed here:

Types, Examples, and Questioning of Thinking Errors

All-or-Nothing Thinking

All-or-nothing thinking is a "black and white" way of thinking. If we think in this way, we only see two choices and no middle ground. This is a common Thinking Error made in thought processes related to healthy eating and physical activity that leads to no attempt at improving or sustaining long-term behavior change.

Examples: "I have just consumed high fat-caloric foods for the past three days, so I might as well splurge until I go back to healthy eating next week"; "If I can't be physically active three to five times per week, why bother doing anything at all!"

Question: What is the middle ground in this situation?

Catastrophizing

We catastrophize when we expect a disastrous or the worst possible outcome from a particular situation. We may also negatively question situational outcomes with "What if?"

Examples: "I'm going to lose all my friends if I quit smoking"; "What if I get fired from my job because no one likes me after I quit smoking?"

Question: How else could the situation turn out?

Disqualifying or Discounting the Positive

When we disqualify or discount the positive we tell ourselves that our positive accomplishments, qualities, or experiences don't hold merit, or aren't worthy of consideration.

Example: "Although I made healthy nutrition choices today, I got lucky because of where I was and the healthy choices I had available to me. I am still undisciplined when it comes to food choices."

Question: What are the positives that I am overlooking?

Mind Reading

We are mind reading when we truly believe we know what others are thinking about us and our capabilities, without consideration of other possibilities that may be more likely.

Example: "Everyone is looking at me at the gym because I am overweight."

Question: Why else might they be acting that way?

"Should" and "Must" Statements

"Should" and "must" statements are common in health behavior change. They occur when we have a set or rigid idea of how we or others should conduct themselves or their behaviors. When our expectations are not met, we negatively overreact.

Example: "What a disaster! I should have never eaten two pieces of sausage pizza! I blew it! I must always eat low-calorie foods!"

Question: Who says it should be this way and why?

Overgeneralization

When we overgeneralize we make "sweeping," overarching negative conclusions that go well beyond the current circumstances or situation.

Example: "I tried the healthy recipes my health coach gave me, but I hated them! I will never like healthy foods! They have no taste whatsoever!"

Questions: When in the past have I tried something that I did not like at first and later enjoyed? Or are there new recipes or healthy cookbooks you can try?

It is important to note that these Thinking Errors can often occur due to our "Core Beliefs."

Core Beliefs are defined as fundamental beliefs or ideas we have about ourselves, the future, others, and the world (Beck, 2011). Our Core Beliefs, accepted as truth or reality, can be positive or negative. The Core Beliefs that need to be challenged and worked on are the ones that are negative and critical in nature. Our past experiences may influence the development of our Core Beliefs and, in turn, impact how we interpret events and our Automatic Thoughts. Automatic Thoughts are situation-specific images or words that go through a person's mind, whereas Core Beliefs are more global in nature.

(Information adapted from J.S. Beck, 2011.)

Core Beliefs

I lead and facilitate training workshops for health and wellness professionals on the application of techniques for health-behavior change. Just today, I followed up with Stacy, one of the outstanding health coaches I trained on behavior change theories last month. Stacy had concerns about a client she has been working with whom she described as being "stuck." Stacy's client, Maria, told her she knew she could not follow through on the things Stacy was asking her to do to improve her recovery from a recent heart attack. Maria had a Core Belief that she could not change her lifestyle behaviors to improve her health status. We all possess Core Beliefs about ourselves and our abilities to change our health behaviors. As the term implies, these beliefs are ingrained in the core of our being. We may have had these beliefs about ourselves for a very long time.

As our Core Beliefs influence our thoughts about ourselves and affect our behaviors on a cognitive level, we must first identify what they are in order to evaluate and self-correct them, if necessary. Maria had been discharged from a rehabilitation facility at a local hospital just days before she began working with Stacy on her health goals. Maria was now faced with the reality that she had to make significant lifestyle changes to prevent further damage to her heart or, even worse, a fatal event next time. Maria was told she had to now take time out of her normally hectic work schedule to go to frequent follow-up appointments with her doctors; significantly reduce her saturated fat and sodium intake; begin a monitored, low-intensity exercise program; and wear a heart monitoring device around the clock. Maria strongly believed that she did not have what it would take to follow through with most of these recommendations her physicians and Stacy gave her. Maria believed she could not succeed and asked Stacy, "If I couldn't make these types of behavior changes in the past, how can I make them now?" Maria revealed her Core Belief in her lack of ability to make positive and necessary health behavior changes. Often we may deal with negative Core Beliefs by either compensating for them or avoiding them altogether. Here, Maria avoided working on her Core Belief in her lack of ability to make positive and necessary behavior changes.

If we hold a Core Belief that we can never lose weight because we have tried and failed so many times, we may believe we are not capable of succeeding, which may subsequently lead to feelings of worthlessness or hopelessness. We may try, again and again, with the same outcome. It is critical for us to first identify our Core Beliefs and change any that will prevent us from making positive behavior changes before attempting to act. Not doing so may result in repeated, fruitless attempts and diminished self-efficacy. In some cases, professional help may be needed if we are trying to change a Core Belief that we have held most of our lives. A professional may help us uncover deeply rooted (or buried) Core Beliefs that we may not be able to uncover on our own. Remember: It is okay—really okay—to ask for help!

Professional help may be obtained from a health care professional trained in psychotherapy, Cognitive Behavioral Therapy (CBT), Motivational Interviewing, or other behavior change theories. In earlier generations, it was a long-standing social norm to equate psychotherapy with severe mental illness. This is no longer the case. It's encouraging that there has been increasing evidence of the acceptance of the social norm of seeking professional help, along with an increase in the utilization of mental health services, as mental and physical health are more simultaneously addressed in a holistic approach to health and wellness. Professional counseling can be especially helpful in changing health behaviors as well as coping with lifecycle changes (Chapter 7).

If you or someone you know is struggling, professional counseling may help expedite negative Core Belief identification, and help confront future situations and events in a constructive and adaptive way to maximize successful health behavior change. Simply picking up the phone and making that first call for help to a properly credentialed and credible professional may make all the difference on your journey toward positive health behavior change. It's important to identify and improve belief modification before behavior modification to optimize your success!

Changing Core Beliefs

If we have identified any negative Core Beliefs related to our abilities to initiate or sustain our desired behavior change, it is important for us to remind ourselves to evaluate them for validity, just like we evaluate our Automatic Thoughts in response to certain situations or events. If a Core Belief is false, we can work to consciously change or modify it. We will want to modify the belief early in the change process, so we can begin to interpret future situations and problems in more constructive and adaptive ways. Modifying a negative Core Belief is a good approach to changing erroneous thinking and beliefs. By modifying a Core Belief to a more realistic belief, one that we can actually believe, we may take smaller but more successful steps toward positive behavior change. If we try to make an extreme change or "stretch" a Core Belief, we will likely not change it because of its potentially questionable validity. Once we have identified and accepted true and positive Core Beliefs about ourselves, we are better prepared for successful health behavior change.

Examples of Modified Core Beliefs

- ↬ Original Core Belief: "I am incompetent when it comes to improving my health habits."

- ↬ New or Modified Core Belief: "I have had both good days and bad when it comes to improving my health habits."

- ↬ Original Core Belief: "I don't have the willpower to stop smoking."

- ↬ New or Modified Core Belief: "I do have control and power over many things in my life. Or, "I do have the willpower to stop smoking for my children."

Emphasize the Positive

"Be self-kind vs. self-critical."
—AMLC

As I am writing this chapter during a much-needed getaway cruise, I am spending time taking care of my well-being and focusing on my thoughts and experiences about changing my health as inspiration for this book. I am also spending precious time with my son, Kyle. Kyle and I love rock and roll music and, as a result, chose this cruise that featured several rock and roll bands. After one of the performances a band offered an open question-and-answer session with the audience. One band member, Jason, was asked by one of the fans in the audience, "What stresses you out?" Jason shared that even after years of doing live-performance shows, he still stresses about his performance after each show. He openly shared that he replays his mistakes, missed notes, and imperfect timing and dance movements. He humbly stated that although he always performed to the best of his ability, he never felt his performance were adequate enough. Surprisingly, Jason is one of the lead members of a very successful and internationally known band. Jason has thousands of loyal followers who love and appreciate his performances and outstanding talents! It saddened me to hear Jason focus on the "negative" aspects of his performances while his audiences did not. Jason discounted the evidence of his abilities by not recognizing the growing number of his fans, along with their positive emotional responses to his performances. This evidence and truth demonstrate that indeed Jason possesses remarkable abilities and is a talented musician!

Of course, it is natural to sometimes focus our thoughts on what we have done wrong, or our mistakes, as opposed to our successes or accomplishments. We sometimes don't see or acknowledge the real truth. This is particularly common among high-achieving individuals (like Jason). When one attains a high level of success in life, he or she may often have very high self-expectations. High self-expectations may fuel one's determination for lifelong, continual self-improvement. As with everything in life, this is not such a bad thing in moderation. However, high-achieving individuals must also be mindful of excessively focusing on the negative aspects of their actions or accomplishments and ignoring the positive. This type of thinking is an example of "disqualifying or discounting the positive." This type of thinking error may negatively affect our Core Beliefs over time.

Any one of us is at risk for not believing in our true selves or in our true abilities if we continuously focus on negative versus positive self-feedback. Over time, emphasis on the negative as opposed to the positive lowers self-efficacy and impedes positive behavior change. Cognitive Behavior Therapy (CBT) employs positive thought processes to improve our mood and behavior. When reflecting upon our reactions to situations, it is important that our thinking be "self-kind" versus "self-critical" to support positive behavior change. Indeed, there is power in positive thinking and positive reflection!

More Tips and Techniques to Change Mindsets

There are several techniques in the literature that have been proven to assist with "changing the way you think about it." A few of the most common are discussed here and others are presented throughout this book. By leveraging these techniques and utilizing your journal, you will be able to identify your thoughts and change any negative thinking to positively change your health!

Credit Lists

An effective technique to evaluate and change or modify false Core Beliefs is to develop "Credit Lists" of both simple as well as challenging accomplishments in a personal journal. Credit Lists also improve self-efficacy and reinforce Mastery Experiences. To develop a Credit List, simply keep a daily list in your journal of all of the healthy behaviors you successfully practiced. Was there something you accomplished in the past that was difficult, but you successfully mastered over time? Credit Lists are useful for reminding us of our successes and accomplishments, and helping us to identify and strengthen our true Core Beliefs. Credit Lists can also serve as visual reminders of our Mastery Experiences and successes we have had throughout our journey toward permanent health behavior change. As on any journey, there may be twists and turns, hills and valleys, and "speed bumps" along the way, but our Credit Lists remind us of our continual progress in the face of life's natural challenges.

Sample Daily Credit List

- I went to the grocery store today to purchase healthy food for the week.
- I completed my "Return to Recess" activity.
- I practiced relaxation techniques.
- I recorded my Automatic Thoughts about a difficult situation in my journal and evaluated them for validity.
- I called the state health department's tobacco "Quit Line" today for help to stop smoking.
- I made an appointment with my doctor today to discuss my ongoing depression.
- I subscribed to a credible diabetes magazine for healthy recipes and tips on managing my diabetes.

Journal Activity

- Develop your Daily Credit List.

Vision Board

A vision board is a tool that can be used to help create clarity and attention to your goals. In today's world, we are overwhelmed with messaging and distractions. It is easy to lose focus on our goals. In addition, we may also fail to clearly identify our goals. There has been some controversy in the field of psychology about the effectiveness of vision boards, but many, including myself, have found them to be an effective way to organize one's goals, values, and dreams, and maintain one's focus in spite of daily distractions.

Vision Board Activity

To create your vision board, get a cardboard or poster board. Look for pictures or postable objects that relate to your health and well-being goals and post them on the board. Hang the board in a visible spot that you view on at least a daily basis. Continually add to your vision board as you are inspired.

Just Say "Later"

Instead of "just saying no" when faced with temptation in your behavior change journey, "just saying later" can assist with self-control. Research has shown that postponing indulging in unhealthy behaviors can help. Putting off the indulgence may be an effective strategy to get past a point of peak desire and, as a result, assist with controlling some behaviors. You can use the process of Counterconditioning (Chapter 2). However, another self-control technique would be to postpone the action. For example, if you are about to reluctantly order an alcoholic beverage, or pick up a cigarette, telling yourself, "I'll have one later" may be an effective technique to temporarily control your behavior. It is a shift from an "impulsive system," evoked by temptation, to a reflective one where we pause, think about the consequences of the action, and re-focus on our goals (Hofman, Friese, and Strack, 2009). Postponing indulgence is another way to change your mind, change your health.

Relaxation

Today's commonly hectic and fast-paced society puts us at risk for negative thought patterns, tension, and stress that can inhibit our progress with positive behavior change. The daily practice of mindfulness, relaxation, and meditation techniques has been shown to reduce these risks. These techniques can help us focus in the present—in the moment—and increase our awareness of physical and emotional sensations without judgment.

Stop, Stretch, and Breathe

In my book, *Winning Health Promotion Strategies* (2010), I describe a program that I developed called "Stop, Stretch, and Breathe," depicted here. Stop, Stretch, and Breathe, as the name implies, is a relaxation program that incorporates deep breathing and stretching. It is a 10-minute routine designed to challenge us to stop at least once a day, stretch our bodies, and breathe with deep, cleansing breaths.

Stop, Stretch, and Breathe

This 10-minute stress management and physical activity program is designed to be performed in a chair. The goal is to increase blood flow, reduce stress, and improve range of motion through stretching, muscle relaxation, and deep breathing.

Stop, Stretch, and Breathe Exercise

You may immediately identify the smell of lavender when you enter the room for your Stop, Stretch, and Breathe session. The sound of water is coming from a small waterfall on a table in the front of the room. The lights are dim, and a screensaver of a fish tank is projected on the front wall of the room. Ocean sounds emanate from a softly playing CD. Take a seat and begin to unwind for a few moments until you begin. Now complete the following steps:

1. Sit up straight and maintain this posture. Let your head balance between your shoulders so no strain is felt in your neck.

2. Close your eyes if you feel comfortable enough to do so. (If not, focus your attention on the screensaver of a fish tank or other relaxing visual projected on the front wall of the room.)

3. Clear your mind, letting go of any stressful, negative, or judgmental thoughts.

4. Notice and focus on your breathing. Your breathing should be slow and fairly regular, without any big gulps of air. Notice

your belly rising as you breathe in through your nose and falling as you breathe out through your mouth.

5. Notice any tightness, soreness, or stiffness in your muscles. Try to relax these muscles by tensing and relaxing them. Notice the difference between tension and relaxation. Now complete five sets each of:

    ~ Deep, relaxing breaths.

    ~ Forward neck rolls.

    ~ Front shoulder rolls.

    ~ Back shoulder rolls.

    ~ Upward shoulder shrugs while breathing in, and breathing out, and releasing tension as shoulders drop.

    ~ Shoulder retractions by pulling shoulders back so that shoulder blades move toward each other.

6. Deeply inhale while raising both arms above head. Hold for a moment, then lower arms slowly while slowly exhaling.

7. Raise one arm, bend to side, and lower slowly. Repeat with other arm.

8. Raise arms overhead again. This time fold forward slowly, lowering your head between your legs until the top your head faces toward the floor. Hold this position for several seconds while continuing to breathe. (This exercise is similar to inverted poses in yoga.)

9. With hands on thighs just above knee caps, come up very slowly with your back in an arched (that is, cat stretch) position.

10. Return to seated position and resume a straight posture.

11. Notice any tense muscles in your body that may remain. If so, tense and relax those muscles until all strain is gone.

12. End session with five deep, relaxing breaths.

Enhancements

~ "Stage" the room with music and appropriate items to enhance relaxation such as scented candles and water fountains.

~~ Add more chair yoga exercises to extend the length of the session.

(Adapted from: *Winning Health Promotion Strategies, Human Kinetics*, 2010)

Deep Breathing

In addition to, or as an alternative to Stop, Stretch, and Breathe, take a few moments throughout a hectic day to simply focus on your breath. Take long, deep, cleansing diaphragmatic (belly) breaths, which are effective for preventing or reducing mental and physical stress and tension. Chest breathing is typically associated with higher levels of mental and physical stress. It is typically shallow, irregular, and sometimes rapid. Belly breathing, however, is associated with deep, slow, and regular breaths. It is the most beneficial breathing technique. Begin by being mindful of your body and breathing. Be still and calm. Inhale deeply, hold for a second, and exhale slowly in a rhythmic way. Deep breathing can be performed at any time or in any place, although it is most effective when sitting or lying down. Each time you exhale, visualize the stress and tension vacating your body. When practicing, place one hand very lightly on your chest, and the other on your belly. If you are breathing correctly, you will feel more movement with the hand on your belly than the hand on your chest. When performed correctly, deep breathing can provide an immediate relaxation response.

Key Points

~~ Automatic Thoughts affect mood and behavior.

~~ Core Beliefs affect behavior change.

~~ It is important to identify and correct Thinking Errors.

~~ Positive thinking improves behavior.

~~ "Just saying later" can assist with immediate self-control.

~~ Practicing relaxation can help improve and manage thoughts and moods.

Action Items

- Monitor, evaluate, and, if necessary, restructure your Automatic Thoughts.
- Keep Thought Records to increase awareness of your thoughts and discover your thought patterns.
- Develop your daily credit list.
- Create your vision board.
- Practice relaxation techniques.

6

Make a New Life Plan

Insider Secret #6:
Lessons From Business School

When I owned a health club, I evaluated its success by examining financial data as well as member outcomes and satisfaction. Usually, the results coincided. My staff and I managed a variety of information and data on a daily, weekly, and monthly basis. We continuously evaluated and managed our financial outcomes related to budgets and projections. I reviewed membership statistics, member progress and results, member satisfaction, program attendance, and utilization of our programs and services. Our goals were achieved when our service quality, member retention and satisfaction, and financial success synergistically came together, resulting in successful experiences for our members as well as positive financial outcomes. We successfully fulfilled our mission when our programs, staff, and facilities were all operating at peak efficiency. Although sometimes challenging to orchestrate, our mission and goals were clear and well-defined in a plan consisting of strategies to achieve and manage them on a daily basis. To maintain a successful business, *a variety of elements needed to be managed throughout a variety of everyday circumstances.* The same is true for behavior change. Just knowing what to do and what not to do about changing our health behaviors isn't enough. Following a clear and well-defined plan, and effectively managing it along with all of life's variables helps us achieve our health goals.

Welcome to the wonderful world of management!

One does not necessarily need to go to business school to become a successful manager. Like other life skills, we can learn effective management techniques and strategies on our own, particularly when we are learning how to self-manage our personal health behaviors. Many individuals embarking on their journey of health behavior change fail because they don't have the necessary *self-management skills* (not to be confused with general management skills) and support systems needed to support a *resilient* habit. Some possess self-management skills and leverage them for other goals, but may not apply them to their goals of health behavior change. In order to achieve improved health behavior outcomes, we need to learn how to be proficient at self-management skills and utilize these skills for health behavior change on a daily basis to be successful.

This chapter will help you identify and develop your self-management and leadership skills as well as utilize your social support systems to successfully change your health behaviors. This chapter will also demonstrate how a clear and well-defined plan to effectively manage behavior change will minimize any potential stress, and maximize motivation and determination. No matter how much we have to juggle in life, sound management principles and practices help us stay organized, stay on target, and maximize successful behavior change.

Management and Leadership

There are notable similarities between managing a business and managing our own health behaviors to include leading, monitoring, organizing, and planning. Let's take a look at these similarities. Management and leadership have similar elements but they are not the same thing. Through the years, there has been much debate over the definition of each. However, most agree that one must possess both management and leadership skills to successfully fulfill a mission, a vision, as well as SMART goals. Whereas management's primary role is to plan, organize, and coordinate, leadership's role is to *motivate and inspire* to excel! Both of these essential skill sets are necessary to "self-manage, self-lead, *and* self-inspire" in order to fulfill one's mission, vision, and SMART goals related to behavior change.

The CEO

"Management Must Manage."
—Harold Geneen

At the "helm," managing, leading, and inspiring every successful local to global organization is a talented chief executive officer (CEO). The CEO is responsible for establishing the mission, the vision, and the goals of the organization; ensuring each and every division or department is being managed effectively and efficiently; and leading and inspiring his or her team to achieve them. A successful and respected CEO effectively manages, leads, and inspires. For personal health behavior change, you are your own CEO. Yes, you! And, like the CEOs of some of the most successful organizations around the world, you have a very important job! Like an organizational CEO must manage the critical operations of divisions or departments, you have to manage all the critical "systems" of your body, such as your skeletal, muscular, nervous, respiratory, cardiovascular, digestive, and immune systems, and so on.

You do this by managing your health behaviors to optimize the functioning of these systems at full capacity throughout the course of your lifetime. As Harold Geneen stated in the previous quote, "Management Must Manage." As self-managers of our health systems and behaviors, we orchestrate, lead, set priorities, set long- and short-term goals, develop an *action* plan, and monitor our progress and adherence to our *action* plan on a daily basis. And, as self-leaders we inspire and motivate ourselves; we become our own cheerleaders! With the proper self-management and self-leadership techniques and strategies, as well as the proper Helping Relationships or social support when needed, we, too, drive our health behaviors for optimal outcomes from the "helm."

As our own personal CEO, we may need to delegate, schedule, problem-solve, strategize, and be able to seamlessly switch gears as necessary to overcome any emerging barriers that may derail our goals and best intentions of accomplishing our mission, vision, and SMART goals related to our health behaviors. We must learn to self-inspire, self-motivate, and self-lead *throughout* our journey of change. Dee Edington, PhD, University of Michigan professor and founder and CEO at Edington Associates, defines self-leadership as "the process of purposefully engaging in change, making thoughtful decisions, and having resilience." Organizational as well as self-leadership takes time, focus, attention, and problem-solving abilities, along with the drive, determination, and grit to succeed.

What Is Your Main Motivation (M²)

For most for-profit businesses the Main Motivation (M²) is financial profit and growth, whether that be by researching, developing, or marketing competitive products or services. For a business to be sustainable and grow over time, it must be profitable. Your M² is the reason *behind* wanting to achieve your goals, or your driving force on this journey of change. What is *your* M²? Do you want to become or stay fit so you can be active with your children? Do you want to live a healthy lifestyle to increase your energy or reduce your depression? Do you want to terminate a problem behavior negatively affecting you or your loved ones? Do you want to lose weight to fit into your wedding dress? If the latter is the case, your *goal* may be to lose weight, but your M² is to do so to fit into your wedding dress, and be fit and radiant on your special day. My M² is to stay fit, healthy, and physically and mentally high functioning for as long as possible throughout the course of an active life. Currently, I am striving to maintain hectic family, work, and travel schedules to continue to do the meaningful work I do, at the pace I need and want to accomplish it. At the same time, I would like to spend quality time with my family, incorporate leisure travel, enjoy outdoor activities such as skiing and biking, and attend rock concerts with my son. These goals motivate me to stay fit and healthy so I can operate at the highest level of physical and mental energy possible to meet the demands of my mission for a fulfilling and thriving life.

Journal Activity

What is your M²? Give some serious consideration and thought to the question. Write your response down and ensure it is really the M² that will drive you to attain and sustain your personal health mission, vision, and SMART goals.

Your Personal Mission and Vision Statements

A good place to begin your behavior change journey as the CEO of your health is to develop a personal mission and vision statement. A mission statement is defined as "a written declaration of an organization's core purpose and focus that normally remains unchanged over time." Your personal mission for your health guides your personal health goals. Properly crafted organizational or personal mission statements (1) serve as filters to separate what is important from what is not; (2) clearly state which "body systems" will be served and how; and (3) communicate a sense of intended direction for your overall health and well-being. A mission is different from a vision in that the former shapes the latter. As you strive to meet your personal mission and vision, your SMART goals may change as you move through the Stages of Change on your journey toward health. Our goals may have to be adaptable or flexible in the face of barriers or adversity, or unpredictable, life-changing or lifecycle events that ebb and flow throughout the course of our lives (Chapter 8). When our health mission and vision serve as filters to separate what is important from what is not, we are able to identify what is most important to focus on, on a daily basis, while communicating a sense of intended direction for our overall health. From a well-defined mission and vision, SMART goals may be set to achieve them.

Developing Your Mission Statement

Your first task as a CEO is to develop a mission statement for your health and well-being. An example of a mission statement is, "As the CEO of my health and well-being, my *mission* statement is to live a happy, healthy, active, and purposeful life."

Journal Activity

As the CEO of your health and well-being, develop your personal mission statement.

Arnold Had a Vision

In his book *100 Ways to Motivate Yourself* (2012), Steve Chandler describes a day in 1977 that he spent with a not-so-well-known Arnold

Schwarzenegger. At the time, Steve was a sports columnist for the *Tucson Citizen* newspaper in Arizona. Arnold was in town to publicize *Stay Hungry*, one of his first movies, and Steve was asked to spend an entire day interviewing Arnold to write a news piece for the Sunday magazine of *Tucson Citizen*. Steve describes his lunch interview with Arnold as the most memorable part of the day. They ate at a restaurant where no one recognized Arnold. During lunch, Steve asked Arnold, "Now that you have retired from bodybuilding, what are you going to do next?" According to Steve, Arnold replied with "a voice as calm as if he were telling me mundane travel plans" and said, "I'm going to be the number-one box office star in all of Hollywood." Listening to Arnold's strong accent and looking at Arnold's huge frame, Steve describes how he was shocked and even amused at Arnold's plan because his first attempt at making movies was not promising. When Steve asked Arnold *just how* he planned on accomplishing this goal, Arnold replied, "It's the same process I used in bodybuilding. What you do is **create a vision** of who you want to be, and then live in that picture as if it was already true." Arnold didn't wait until he "received a vision." He created one. And, the rest is history....

Developing Your Vision Statement

Your second task as a CEO is to develop a vision statement for your health and well-being. A sample vision statement is, "As the CEO of my health and well-being, my *vision* statement is to thrive by living my life with health and vitality in order to be able to fulfill my hopes and dreams."

Journal Activity

As the CEO of your health and well-being, develop your personal vision statement.

Breaking Down Your Mission Statement Into Core Elements

Breaking down your mission statement in a list of Core Elements and tasks that will help you achieve your mission is very helpful. Following is a sample list of Core Elements and associated tasks that will help me achieve my personal mission statement: *to live a **happy**, **healthy**, active, and **purposeful** life.*

Core Elements

Happy

- Spend more quality, relaxed, fun times with my husband, son, and family.
- Remember and reflect on fond memories of late loved ones by making scrapbooks and photo books, visiting the cemetery, and praying.
- Travel for leisure with my husband and son.
- Spend time relaxing with close friends.
- Play with my pets.
- Enjoy music, listen to my old vinyl records, and attend concerts with my son.
- Spend time alone at a beach or spa, reading a good book, or just relaxing.
- Pray and practice gratitude in my daily life.

Healthy

- Nourish my body daily with healthy foods and adequate water intake.
- Be physically active daily, including Return to Recess.
- Manage my stress through meditation or other relaxation techniques.
- Maximize quality sleep by managing my schedule and ensuring I get enough "downtime" and rest.
- Keep up-to-date on my routine and annual exams (for example, primary care provider, dentist, cancer screenings, and so on).

Active

- Enjoy and engage in outdoor activities such as skiing throughout my most active years and into my senior years.
- Continue an active pace of work *and* a leisure lifestyle.

- Travel to the places on my "wish list" before and into my golden years.

Purposeful

- Engage in projects or work that provides me with sense of meaning and helps me and others to *thrive*.
- Mentor the next generation in the health and wellness field.
- Help those in need.

Journal Activity

Review your personal mission statement, and break it down into a list of Core Elements and tasks that will help you achieve it.

Prioritization

After you have made the list of your Core Elements and associated tasks to achieve your personal mission, prioritize the Core Elements or areas of your mission statement you are ready to begin changing. Concentrate on the areas in which you are in a stage of readiness to change (for example, *contemplation* or *preparation*). It is important to not only focus on your priority areas or those most important to you to begin your journey of change, but also those areas that present the fewest barriers to change. *Every* CEO has to prioritize. It is very difficult to provide the focus and attention to all areas of your health and well-being simultaneously while balancing your work life, home life, and unpredictable lifecycle events. It is important to be realistic as you determine and begin addressing your priorities. Once you have prioritized your list of Core Elements and associated tasks, it is time to set SMART goals to achieve your overall mission.

Goal-Setting

> *"A man without a goal is like a ship without a rudder."*
> —Thomas Carlyle

As Thomas Carlyle implies, and as Earl Nightingale once said, "Without a goal, one's mission and vision cannot be guided and may become subject to any shift in direction due to changes in wind, tides, currents, or anything else posing threat to reaching a 'destination.'" Clear and well-defined goals provide focus and direction. Goals serve as the "rudder" needed to keep on course, without detours, to reach a destination as quickly and directly as possible. Once you have gone through the steps of prioritizing the Core Elements and associated tasks of your mission statement, you may then set SMART Goals to achieve each Core Element.

SMART Goal-Setting

Goal-setting is a critical component of successful behavior change. Goals, tailored to Stage of Change and level of self-efficacy, must be set. Effective goal-setting will maximize opportunities for successful health behavior change (Hobbis *et al.*, 2005). By writing our goals in a journal, we are giving thoughtful attention to our change processes.

SMART goals are those that are *Specific, Measurable, Attainable, Realistic, and Time-based.* Goal-setting helps one work toward meeting his or her own objectives, and is featured as a major component in the literature on personal development and behavior change. The term *goal* is one of the most recognizable words in motivational management. As goals or components of goals are accomplished or new discoveries are made, goals may be modified for continual progress toward one's ultimate mission. Studies have shown that ambitious goals may lead to a higher level of performance than less challenging goals, but to optimize successful achievement, goals must be *Attainable* and *Realistic* as well. SMART Goals motivate us to set our own standards for self-satisfaction with performance (Olson, Schmidt, Winkler. and Wipfli, 2011).

Specific

Set a Specific goal for the behavior you would like to change. For example, instead of saying you would like to lose weight, specify *how much* (I want to lose 10 pounds, 20 pounds, 50 pounds).

Measureable

Make certain your goals are Measurable. Weight-loss progress may be measured with a scale, or the circumference of your waist, hips, and so on. Attainment of goals related to healthy eating or improved nutrition may be measured by monitoring food intake with a food diary or 24-hour dietary recall; progress toward physical activity, sleep, and other goals may be measured by keeping a daily activity log, using "apps," or the Internet, or with wearable technology tracking devices.

Attainable

Ensure the goals you set are Attainable and based on your current Stage of Change, or "where you are at" now.

Realistic

Base your goals on a Realistic assessment of your time commitment, barriers, and supports to changing a behavior, and other influencing variables in your life.

Time-based

Set a time frame for your goals. For example, national guidelines recommended a weight-loss goal of no more than two pounds per week. If your goal is to lose 10 pounds, a Time-based (and Realistic) goal would be to lose 10 pounds within the next 45 days, not in one week.

Short-Term and Long-Term SMART Goals

SMART goals may be short-term or long-term. Short-term goals are setting expectations for achievements or accomplishments in a relatively shorter period of time. An example of a short-term goal may be to cut down from 10 to two cigarettes per day throughout the course of four weeks, or complete your Commitment Contract to Return to Recess (Chapter 3) for a week. A short-term goal may be set to be accomplished on a daily, weekly, or monthly basis. Long-term goals may be set to be accomplished throughout several months or longer. For example, if your goal was to lose 25 pounds of excess weight, this goal could be set to be accomplished over a period of three to six months or longer.

Journal Activity

Categorize your SMART goals to achieve the Core Elements in your mission statement by whether or not they are short-term or long-term.

Developing a Plan

> "If you fail to plan, you are planning to fail!"
> —Benjamin Franklin

Once you have determined your mission and vision, identified the Core Elements of your mission, and set your short- and long-term SMART goals to accomplish them, you have developed the "framework" of your individualized plan for health behavior change! When you develop and follow your personalized, written plan, you strategically position yourself for success. Your plan is your "blueprint" or "road map" that includes the path or direction you will need to take on your journey to change to get to your "destination." For example, if one of your short-term SMART goals is healthy eating, you need to detail out all the steps needed to achieve your goal, including supportive or enhanced activities for accomplishing this goal. These steps may include leveraging the appropriate processes of change (Chapter 2), additional strategies throughout this book, developing and sticking to a weekly food plan, shopping for healthy foods, gathering healthy recipes, and scheduling a session with a nutritionist (many supermarkets now offer free sessions with registered dietitians or nutritionists).

If one of your long-term SMART goals is to gradually increase your level of physical activity over six months, you may plan to leverage the appropriate processes of change (Chapter 2), along with other strategies throughout this book, keep a daily physical activity log, research and purchase new or used home fitness equipment, hire a personal trainer, and seek out pertinent and credible resources on the Internet. In the "app age," there are numerous applications available for you to use on your electronic devices to track and monitor your behavior change activities and progress. You may also use your journal *daily* to plan and log your dietary intake and physical activity, as well as document any personal thoughts and circumstances along your journey toward positive and permanent health behavior change.

Daily Tracking and Monitoring of Your Plan

Tracking and monitoring your plan daily is a bit like performing a daily analysis of business activity. If you develop a weekly plan, track and monitor how much progress you are making on a daily basis to gauge where you are and where you are headed in relation to your goals and mission. Plan, track, and monitor your activities and progress toward achieving your goals. Don't leave your progress to chance.

Journal Activity

Develop a written plan, and track and monitor your progress, mission, and goals on a daily basis. If necessary, make necessary adjustments. Note any barriers, challenges, or other circumstances that arose, along with how you overcame these situations.

Overcoming Barriers and Problem-Solving

As the personal CEO of our health and well-being, we must be able to identify any potential challenges or barriers that may be standing in the way of achieving our mission, vision, and SMART goals. Once we identify barriers or challenges, we need to identify possible solutions to successfully overcome them. Sound easy? Sometimes, it is not. Over the course of 10 years that I operated my health club, I worked with thousands of members. I was surprised at how many people, including myself, had difficulty actually identifying the *real* barriers holding them back from making positive health behavior change. Previously I described my story about my "jet set" lifestyle and how I justified my poor health choices. My own personal denial of the true barriers holding me back from healthy eating on the constant run and "up in the air" kept me from clearly identifying my barriers and, in turn, overcoming them by brainstorming solutions. For successful behavior change, it is important to learn how to differentiate between real and perceived barriers. On our journeys of behavior change, any one of us may experience barriers that surface at one time or another. Whether real or perceived, barriers come between us and our goals. In order to successfully overcome them, we first need to identify them, and then determine whether they are real or perceived. Only then can we overcome or break through them by developing alternative strategies to achieve positive behavior change.

The 10 most common reasons adults cite for not adopting more physically active lifestyles are listed here (Sallis and Hovell, 1990; Sallis, Hovell, and Hofstetter 1992). These barriers are currently listed on Centers for Disease Control and Prevention (CDC) Website (2011) and remain problematic more than a decade later. Also listed are sample solutions to each of these 10 barriers (and others). Check out the CDC website for a more comprehensive listing of solutions to overcoming them.

The 15 Most Common Reasons for Physical Inactivity and Sample Solutions

1. Do not have enough time to exercise.
   - Multi-task and exercise while watching the news.
   - Return to Recess or exercise in short bouts that fit into your schedule.
   - Replace a sedentary activity, such as watching television or going online, with alternative options (for example, taking your dog for a walk).
   - Delegate other things you need to do to fit exercise into your day.

2. Find it inconvenient to exercise.
   - Explore simple ways to make it convenient for you, such as traveling with an exercise band, or putting a piece of visible exercise equipment in your living room and using it as you watch your favorite television show.

3. Lack self-motivation.
   - Leverage the many tips and techniques throughout this book to enhance your motivation.
   - Continually refer to your vision statement to "fuel your fire" to persevere and achieve your mission and SMART goals!

4. Do not find exercise enjoyable.
   - Complete your Activity History to identify activities that you find enjoyable.
   - Leverage Return to Recess strategies and techniques to make it fun (Chapter 3)!
   - Exercise with a friend to enhance the enjoyment of moving!

5. Find exercise boring.
   - Motivate yourself by starting with Return to Recess.
   - Explore the many different ways you may incorporate physical activity or movement into your daily schedule.

- Find what you enjoy most by "sampling" different options.

6. Lack confidence in the ability to be physically active (low self-efficacy).

   - Complete the Self-Efficacy Activity and leverage the four sources to overcome this barrier for good (Chapter 4).

7. Fear being injured or experienced recent injury.

   - Check with your physician before beginning any exercise program.

   - If you have been injured recently or fear a recurring injury, seek advice from a healthcare professional (for example, a physical therapist).

8. Lack self-management skills, such as the ability to set personal goals, monitor progress, or reward progress toward such goals.

   - Leverage the strategic planning tips and techniques presented in this chapter.

   - Develop a written plan, and track and monitor your daily progress, challenges, and circumstances in your journal.

   - Reward yourself with healthy rewards as you reach the milestones of your SMART goals (for example, massage, spending time in nature or with loved ones, or just a day of simple day or evening of "downtime").

9. Lack encouragement, support, or companionship from family and friends.

   - Seek encouragement and support from support groups, or other groups offered at community-based organizations (for example, churches, community hospitals, or health clubs).

   - Seek immediate support as well as lasting relationships with those with similar behavior change goals from credible community-based and online support groups for the behavior(s) you are seeking to change. Talk openly with family or friends about your goals and how they might be able to support you.

10. Lack parks, sidewalks, bicycle trails, or safe and pleasant walking paths convenient to home or office.

    ~ Drive to convenient parks in the area.

    ~ Utilize large shopping malls for walking (particularly in inclement weather).

11. Costly programs.

    ~ Check for free or low-cost programs at your community recreation department, senior center, or community hospital.

    ~ Find out if your employer's health insurer (or financial investment company) offers health and wellness programs.

    ~ Search the Internet for credible and free/low-cost resources and programs.

12. Poor-quality programs that are weak in content, instruction, or not fun (or all three).

    ~ Explore different programs until you discover high quality options that meet your needs and expectations.

13. Programs requiring use of technology that may be stress-provoking in individuals without proficiency.

    ~ Seek programs without technology components (for example, your state or local health department's telephonic smoking cessation or "quit line").

    ~ Check for non-technology-related, in-person programs offered by your health plan or through your local community.

14. Lack of energy or motivation.

    ~ Ensure you are getting enough sleep and proper nutrition.

    ~ Keep your stress levels low.

- ☙ If you have experienced long-term fatigue, talk to your physician. He or she may recommend a depression, thyroid, and/or vitamin D screening.
- ☙ If lack of motivation is the issue at hand, leverage the strategies and techniques presented throughout this book to give your motivation a boost!

15. Cultural and language barriers.

- ☙ Check for cultural organizations in your community that know, understand, and support your cultural practices and needs. Ask what resources they would recommend.
- ☙ Check with your medical plan or physician for information on culturally appropriate health resources in multiple languages.

(Adapted from *Winning Health Promotion Strategies*, Ludovici-Connolly, 2010.)

Successful adoption of behavior change requires the ability to identify and overcome barriers to change. The more skilled you become at early identification and reduction of your barriers to change, the better chance you have at achieving your goals of health behavior change. Although many of the barriers and sample solutions listed pertain to physical activity, most apply to other health behaviors as well. As your personal CEO, once you identify the barriers to your success, you can then begin to strategize your personalized solutions to overcome them.

Journal Activity

List all of your perceived barriers to improving the health behavior you want to change. For each barrier, list possible *solutions* to overcome it.

Time Management

"If you don't manage your time, it will manage you."
—Annie

As a consultant for a national health and wellness firm, my colleagues and I were required to track our work activity every 15 minutes.

This may seem a bit excessive, however, it was one of the best exercises I was ever required to do at work! Due to the fact that I worked on several different client projects at one time, I needed to report exactly what I was spending my time on to accurately bill our clients. This exercise also was extremely helpful to me as I strove to optimally and appropriately manage my time. I began each day scheduling my projects and associated work tasks, including conference calls with clients. To this day, as I continue to provide consultative services, I track my activities every quarter hour throughout my workday. This keeps me on track and allows me to be most productive by not wasting time on frivolous tasks. As I keep track of my time on scheduled tasks, I am less likely to be distracted or "pulled away" from priority projects. I establish my weekly and daily schedules to include time devoted to my Return to Recess as well as other SMART goals I have set to achieve my overall health mission.

Lack of time is one of the most common barriers cited for successful health behavior change. If you don't keep track of and manage your time, lack of time will surely be a barrier that will keep you from achieving your goals for behavior change. One need not manage every 15 minutes of every day to effectively manage time. However, it is one helpful strategy to evaluate how one spends the majority of his or her time, some of which could possibly be managed more efficiently to achieve priority goals for behavior change. In addition to my daily journal where I tracked my dietary intake, physical activity, personal thoughts, and circumstances, I maintain a calendar with scheduled tasks in my day planner in order to achieve and maintain my health goals. I have colleagues and clients who don't track every 15 minutes of their workday, but they keep a daily calendar to schedule their priorities to help them keep on track with their mission, vision, and SMART goals. Almost all mobile devices have scheduling applications with prompts and notifications to stay on task. Explore these or other strategies for scheduling, tracking, and monitoring that may work for you.

Delegation

Carol, a client of mine, is a mom, wife, daughter, and busy executive. She felt she had no time to devote to improving her health. We sat down and worked together on her mission statement. Carol defined her vision, established SMART goals, identified her barriers, reprioritized her health, and developed a personalized plan. As a business executive proficient in delegation, Carol realized a primary way for her to reduce her barrier of lack of time was to delegate some of her routine tasks in her life to free up time to devote to improving her health and well-being.

Carol and I began by making a list of all of the tasks she had to routinely accomplish to keep her household operating. Carol then identified which of those tasks could be delegated. Some of the items on Carol's delegation list included:

- House cleaning.
- Grocery shopping.
- Running errands (for example, dry cleaner, pharmacy, bank, tailor).
- Cooking meals.
- Picking up kids at school and taking them to after-school activities and events.

Delegation, a fundamental management principle, can be an effective skill to assist with freeing up time to accomplishing your goals for behavior change, without neglecting other priorities that could possibly result in stress and negative consequences.

Journal Activity

- Make a list of your routine tasks or chores that you need to do.
- Identify which of your routine tasks or chores that you may be able to delegate.
- Identify *who* you can speak to regarding the delegation of specific tasks.

Effective Delegation

When Carol began delegating, she had identified her 18-year-old son, John, as a perfect choice to do the weekly grocery shopping for the family. John had a driver's license, he was at an age where he was taking on more family responsibilities, and he had some free time because his job had cut back his hours. Although new and awkward to John at first (and frustrating to Carol), he quickly learned how to select the correct supermarket items, brands, and sizes used by his family.

Tips for Effective Delegation

- ❧ Delegate the right tasks to the right people.
- ❧ Be clear and specific with your needs and instructions.
- ❧ Communicate what, when, where, and how you need tasks accomplished.

If you are a perfectionist, be willing to "let go." Despite the old adage "If you want something done right, do it yourself," efficient and effective CEOs realize they can't do everything themselves. They know how to hire the right people, lead, inspire, teach, and *delegate* for success. They know how to provide "over the shoulder support" when needed. After Carol's initial frustration with the items John initially purchased at the grocery store, Carol realized she did not provide him with enough direction to complete the task successfully. Her Automatic Thoughts were "My son won't be able to do this. I will just have to keep doing it by myself." Carol and I discussed how we could re-structure her Automatic Thought, and she changed her thought to "Maybe he can do this with a bit of initial support." Carol decided to go with John to the grocery store the following week, and clearly and specifically communicated her needs and instructions. She taught him exactly what she wanted, the "what, when, where, and how." When John went alone the following week, he purchased everything on the list, exactly what Carol wanted.

Start with small steps. Carol could have employed another strategy when delegating the weekly grocery shopping to John. She could have started with delegating a smaller list with weekly and gradual increases in the size of list as John's "self-efficacy" improved and Carol improved her communication skills. When delegation of a task is unsuccessful, try delegating a different one. Even after clear and specific communication of needs and instructions, John may not have been a "good fit" for the specific task of grocery shopping per Carol's expectations. If that had been the outcome, Carol could have easily delegated a different task to John, such as running other weekly household errands.

Make an Investment

If you are in a financial position to purchase services or pay someone to help you, it may be worth the investment to eliminate the barrier of lack of time. For example, if you don't have anyone to delegate the task of grocery shopping to, consider home delivery services. Other purchasable services include house cleaning, assistance with weekly errands, and so on.

Combining Tasks

In Steve Chandler's book *100 ways to Motivate Yourself* (2012), he describes how we can delegate activities, but also combine activities that support our goals. In order to simplify his life, Chandler describes how he combined the task of grocery shopping with spending time with his children, one of his personal goals related to his overall health and well-being. Sometimes you can "combine" your mission, vision, and SMART goals. For example, perhaps someone in your community or church needs yard work. You could help someone and, at the same time, focus on your health and well-being objectives by getting some additional physical activity and helping someone in need.

Journal Activity

List any tasks or activities you can combine to achieve your mission, vision, and SMART goals to fulfill your plan for behavior change.

Saving Progress to Get Ahead, Not to Break Even

One of my previous health club members, Jan, monitored her weight weekly as recommended. She admitted to occasionally thinking if she lost one to two pounds one week, she could eat larger portions or indulge in her favorite desserts the following week. By doing so, Jan was not achieving her weight-loss goal. Every time she would make progress, she would "spend" her calories undoing the work she had accomplished during the previous week. We can think of our progress with behavior change as a financial investment. If we "save money in the bank" by making progress, we can let that money reap the cumulative effects of positive behavior change. On the flip side of the coin, we can spend our progress and simply break even. To *get ahead* or make progress with whatever lifestyle behavior change we are working on, we must learn to build a "net savings" over time.

Key Points

- Self-management *and* self-leadership are critical to for successful behavior change.
- *You* are the CEO of your health and well-being.
- Developing a mission and vision statement provides focus and direction.
- Setting SMART goals provides a clear course of action.
- Developing and implementing your behavior change plan will set achievement of your SMART goals into *action*.
- Identify solutions to barriers early to maximize your success.
- Manage your time so it won't manage you!
- Learn to delegate to make more time to focus on implementing your behavior change plan.

Action Items

- Develop your mission and vision statements.
- List and prioritize the Core Elements of your mission statement.
- Set short-term and long-term SMART goals to accomplish your mission.
- Develop your plan.
- Schedule your time and stick to your schedule.
- Continuously track and monitor your progress.
- Make adjustments to your plan, as needed, for success!

7

Game On!

Insider Secret #7:
Power Strategies From Sports Psychology

"Most athletes and coaches will acknowledge that at least 40 to 90 percent of the success in sport is due to mental factors. On a competitive level, it is not uncommon to hear that the winner invariably comes down to who is the strongest athlete— mentally—on a given day!"
—J.M. Williams and V. Krane

As I mentioned earlier, I was privileged to work with several of the teams who were competing in the 1982 America's Cup races. Like all professional athletes, these crew members have physical talents many people lack, but what really sets them apart are their incredible mental strength, internal motivation, and undying determination. One may think that mental strength, motivation, and determination are innate qualities, but there were days these fit, world-class athletes *did not* want to work out. On those days, the crew members used a variety of motivational strategies used in the field of sports psychology, such as vividly declaring their need, and want, to keep their competitive edge to *win*. They used motivational cue phrases and affirmations like *"We gotta keep our EDGE!* At the time, I was in awe over the mental stamina of these athletes. I have since learned that world-class athletes commonly train mentally almost as much as they train physically. Mental training enables them to overcome inevitable obstacles to achieving goals. Winners train to *get* motivated and *stay* motivated, no matter what.

Studies in neuropsychology have proven that affirmations have a positive effect on performance. Psychological techniques for motivation have been used in sports and exercise for more than five decades. Many competitive athletes routinely consult with sports psychologists, who do not prescribe performance-enhancing supplements, but something much more powerful: techniques of the *mind*. Because lack of motivation is a common primary reason given for dropping out of health and wellness programs, this chapter presents a variety of highly effective strategies and techniques adapted from sports and exercise psychology that may be used on your own. They have been shown to motivate even the most demotivated individuals, and sustain motivation in others during times when it is most likely to lag. So, let's get right into some of these techniques that you can leverage to "jump start" your motivation to change and implement your plan for successful behavior change!

Let's begin by exploring the theory of mental toughness. Mental toughness is defined as "a multifaceted construct made up of multiple key components including values, attitudes, cognitions, emotions, and behaviors that refer to an individual's ability to thrive through both positively and negatively construed challenges, pressures, and adversities" (Gucciardi, Gordon, and Dimmock, 2009, p. 64). The America's Cup crews most notably demonstrate their abilities for mental toughness, focus, concentration, confidence, motivation, and their ability to thrive under pressure and in the face of a multitude of setbacks and barriers. One may adopt attributes of mental toughness to the Core Elements of his or her mission and personal behavior change goals to benefit from the "consequences of mental toughness." H.R. Cox, Y. Qiu, and Z. Liu (1993) present 13 attributes of mental toughness:

1. Self-confident along with high self-efficacy.
2. Ability to laser focus and intensely concentrate.
3. Intrinsically motivated.
4. Strong work ethic.
5. Committed to excellence.
6. Persistent and self-determined.

7. Positive attitude.

8. Resilient in the face of failure or injury.

9. Thrive under pressure and challenge.

10. Consistent personal values.

11. Emotional intelligence.

12. Physical toughness.

13. Gracious in the face of success.

Let's explore some of the attributes of mental toughness, as well as sports psychology techniques that can be applied on our journey of behavior change. Many of the other attributes listed are also included in the elements of positive psychology and well-being that will be revealed in later chapters.

Intrinsic Motivation

Reinforcement Management or rewards, recognition, and other incentives for participation in health behavior change programs can be very effective strategies for health behavior change. Financial incentives can be effective in *later* Stages of Change (Chapter 2), when we are ready to take action or maintaining our goals. Reinforcement and recognition can assist us in earlier stages, and throughout the change process, to improve our self-efficacy through verbal persuasion. Rewards and recognition are classified as forms of *external* motivation. External or "extrinsic" motivation, as the word indicates, is rewards or feedback that is received from external sources. Examples include financial incentives for participating in employee wellness programs (or financial penalties for not participating), recognition, praise, awards, and other forms of rewards and recognition that come from external sources. If we are in *earlier* Stages of Change, it is critical to develop "intrinsic" motivation to begin our journey of change. As we continue to make progress, and in later stages of change, intrinsic motivation will help *sustain* progress, overcome setbacks and relapses, and *successfully* help us move forward in our health behavior change journey.

> *"The kind of motivation that exhibits the highest level of self-determination, autonomy, and agency is referred to as being intrinsic or internal in nature."*
> —R.H. Cox

Throughout my career, I have witnessed individuals reaching *action* and sustaining *maintenance* and *termination*. These individuals who successfully implemented and *sustained* their plan for health behavior change had one thing in common: a high level of intrinsic motivation. Most importantly, they were able to sustain their intrinsic motivation over time and adapt through the "chutes and ladders" and "lifecyle" changes of life (Chapter 8). Those with a high level of intrinsic motivation demonstrate the ability to be resilient in the face of adversity, "failure," physical injuries, or other setbacks. Achieving a high level of intrinsic motivation is not easy, but it is achievable. Once achieved, one must work at maintaining it until it becomes an innate quality supportive of permanent behavior change. Individually appealing goals and related tasks help us achieve a higher level of intrinsic motivation. For this reason, it is important that we choose programs to support our goals for health behavior change that we find interesting, fun, and most likely to intrinsically motivate us.

There are three dimensions of intrinsic motivation:

1. Motivation toward knowledge.
2. Motivation toward accomplishment.
3. Motivation toward experiencing stimulation.

Motivation Toward Knowledge

No matter what Stage of Change we are currently in, to improve our intrinsic motivation, we must have a thirst for knowledge for the health behavior we have and fuel a desire to change. As Francis Bacon's quote reminds us, "Knowledge is Power." This quote can easily be applied to intrinsic motivation as well as assist us in early Stages of Change. The more motivated we are to learn about strategies or ways to change our behavior on an ongoing basis, the more likely we are to strengthen our intrinsic motivation. Even if we think we already know what we need to do to achieve our behavior change goals, there is always room to learn more! An ongoing and insatiable thirst for knowledge intrinsically motivates us while propelling us forward to *action* and keeps us in *maintenance* and *termination*. Successful athletes continually drive themselves to learn more and more about their game, their personal performance, and how to improve their competitive edge. They use the process of Consciousness Raising when evaluating their own performance, strengths, and opportunities for improvement, even in the face of potential barriers (Chapter 2). By continuously striving to acquire new skills and learn different and diverse ways to approach all types of situations to accomplish their goals, they reach a higher level of performance. If we adopt this same motivation toward knowledge and learning, we, too, can intrinsically motivate ourselves to accomplish the mission and goals of our own behavior change maintained throughout the course of our lifetimes!

Motivation Toward Accomplishment

> *"Intrinsic motivation toward accomplishment reflects an athlete's desire to gain mastery over a particular skill and the pleasure that comes from reaching a personal goal for mastery."*
> —R.H. Cox

"Building Confidence Through Mastery" (Chapter 4) described how mastery experiences build self-efficacy. Building on and celebrating our successes and mastery experiences, including the "small" successes, simultaneously builds our sense of accomplishment and intrinsic motivation. In earlier Stages of Change, we may have a low level of intrinsic motivation. That is perfectly okay! Behavior change may start off at a slow pace, but improves over time with our self-efficacy and intrinsic motivation. The self-efficacy scale helps us to monitor and maximize our confidence in achieving our priority health behavior changes (Chapter 4). The more efficacious we are, the more motivated we are for accomplishment and self-achievement. This tenacity also minimizes our perceived barriers to reaching our "end zone."

Motivation Toward Experiencing Stimulation

Motivation toward experiencing stimulation is also reflective of what drives an individual to accomplish a specific goal or task. This stimulation may be a physical or emotional sensation, or a rush of adrenaline, from successful achievement of one's goal. Like Dramatic Relief, this is a powerful dimension that increases intrinsic motivation (Chapter 2). With repeated success, one can develop a craving for a feeling of accomplishment.

I often ask people how they feel after being physically active, practicing meditation, or walking away from an alcoholic drink or any other type of temptation they may be trying to avoid; they report feeling *empowered!* The mental and physical stimulation from the feelings of accomplishment are maximized with intrinsic motivation. So, just go for it!

Mental Practice

"Before every shot I go to the movies inside my head.
Here is what I see. First, I see the ball where I want it to finish,
nice and white and sitting up high on the bright green grass.
Then, I see the ball going there; its path and trajectory and even
its behavior on landing. The next scene shows me making the
kind of swing that will turn the previous image into a reality.
These home movies are a key to my concentration and to my
positive approach to every shot."
—Jack Nicklaus

As this golf great Jack Nicklaus's quote describes, many athletes from all sports mentally rehearse or practice their motor skills and movements on a daily basis as well as moments before an event. The literature describes "mental practice" as a form of athletic practice to be equally important as physical practice. Nicklaus stated that a good golf shot is based on 10 percent swing, 40 percent stance and setup, and 50 percent mental preparation for how the swing should occur (Weinberg and Gould, 2011). Imagine that!

One morning, as I walked into the fitness center at the Newport Athletic Club, Jon, the "grinder" for America's boat "Defender," was sitting on the floor straddling and peddling a lifecycle with his hands and arms (as opposed to his feet and legs). The grinder is responsible for hoisting the sails, pulling the winches in, letting them out, and bringing them down. The grinder has the most physically demanding job on the boat. So much so that the grinder is often referred to as sailing's equivalent of a football lineman. Jon was both physically and mentally strong and determined!

Another team member, Mike, sitting on the seat of the lifecycle, varied the intensity on the lifecycle's control panel for Jon, still sitting on the floor. Jon yelled out commands to his teammate to increase the intensity, such as "Give me more!" Jon was attempting to replicate the exact movements and motions of his position on the boat for a couple of reasons. One, Jon wanted "specificity" to train his specific muscles that would be activated for specific repetitive movements needed to hoist the sails. Two, as was very evident, Jon was mentally rehearsing or practicing for the race. Jon closed his eyes, gritted his teeth, and sweat up a storm. I could see that Jon was mentally visualizing himself on the boat in the water. He was going through the exact motions and movements and intensities that he needed to perform on the boat. Jon mentally rehearsed his performance for the entire race.

It is common for athletes to walk through every detail of their performance prior to competitions. Mental rehearsal of competitive events enables athletes to more confidently perform during the actual event.

Defining Mental Practice

Several different terms have been used to describe mental practice, such as imagery, mental rehearsal, and visualization. These terms refer to mentally creating or re-creating experiences. Regardless of whatever term is used, the process begins by recalling from memory, experience, or observational pieces of information. This information may be used to shape these pieces together into meaningful, relevant images (Weinberg and Gould, 2011). Ideally, mental practice involves as many senses as possible. The more one can create images that are vivid and real, the more powerful the technique is at creating an emotional response. Jon, the grinder for the America's Cup, leveraged multiple senses in his mental practice. With a vivid imagination, Jon re-created his kinesthetic sense by moving his body in the specific positions he would need to use on the boat. Leveraging his auditory senses, he imagined hearing the sound of the sails snap as the boat tacked and his teammates yelled commands. He peddled with his arms and hands with all his might. He mentally practiced every tactical approach, including when and how he would perform each task. Jon may have even imagined the smell of the ocean, the spray of salt water on his face, and the wind whipping through his long blonde hair. Re-creating emotional responses and thoughts is also an important part of mental practice. For example, emotional responses such as anger, pain, joy, and anxiety, or thoughts such as lack of confidence or loss of concentration, may positively or negatively impact mental practice. Imagery is a form of stimulation or emotional arousal. If performed correctly, the result is equivalent to a real sensory and mental experience.

Applying Mental Practice to Your Health Behavior

The application of mental practice to health behavior change is a "hidden gem." Think about how you can apply this technique to achieving your health goals. For example, if one of your goals is to exercise at a health club on your walk home from work, you can rehearse the entire process during your walk. Imagine yourself arriving, entering the club, removing your workout clothes from your gym bag, putting them on, and closing your locker. Visualize the piece of equipment you will exercise on and go through your entire workout in your mind. Engage all your senses in the entire experience. Hear the music playing, feel your body and muscles move, smell the soap in the locker room. Imagine getting through the first five minutes of your warm-up, then getting to the 15-minute mark, and then the exhilaration you feel at the 25-minute mark when your endorphins kick in, and your sense of accomplishment during your five-minute cool-down. Imagine how invigorated you feel afterward.

Mental practice will increase your engagement in your workout or *any* other health behavior, and will put you more at ease or on "automatic pilot" to optimize success. If you are in *action* for smoking cessation, mentally practice from the time you wake up in the morning and "walk" through your day using Counterconditioning techniques, monitoring your Automatic Thoughts, and using verbal cues, mindfulness, and other strategies to keep you on track until you go to sleep (chapters 2 and 5). If you know you will be at an event that evening where others may be smoking, mentally go through the steps that you will take to minimize the temptation to smoke. Visualize every potential sensory experience of the event: the lights, the sounds, the taste of the food served, even the smell of cigarette smoke when you enter or exit the building. Imagine a positive or healthy response to all stimuli. Be mindful, and mentally practice how you will deal with any challenging situations so you will stay on course to reach your endzone!

Lucy the Cheetah

Lucy suffered from stress and mild depression and lacked energy for quite some time. Because Lucy was in good physical health, her physician wanted her to get more physical activity before prescribing any depression medication. Lucy agreed and came to me to begin a program. We worked on several techniques that she could leverage to get started. We discussed Lucy's sleep patterns, and nutrition, and how she was currently managing her stress and depression. Together we discovered that Lucy's main barrier to being physically active was fatigue brought on by her mild depression. Because Lucy was not motivated to get physically active as her physician recommended, we set one of her goals to be engaging in Return to Recess on a daily basis. I also demonstrated some stress-management techniques that Lucy practiced with me. One technique that Lucy found particularly helpful was "Energizing Imagery." We discussed all the different scenarios and images that Lucy could choose from that "energized" her to help her push through her fatigue. She chose to imagine herself as a cheetah. Lucy always had a fascination with cheetahs and what they represented (strength, grace, power, and a robust amount of energy).

Ironically, Lucy learned that the cheetah can run faster than any other land animal on earth! As Lucy closed her eyes and took deep relaxing breaths, she imagined herself as a cheetah, running at a steady pace through tall grasslands. After 30 minutes of practicing Energizing Imagery, Lucy shared with me all of the imagery and sensations she experienced. Lucy exclaimed, "I never felt more energized!" At our next visit, I presented Lucy with a little stuffed cheetah that would serve as a visual prompt to remind Lucy that she always had the power within her to go back to that time and place, *wherever* she was. Over time, by *changing her mind*, Lucy *changed her health* by becoming physically active, which alleviated her depression. What a wonderful experience to witness Lucy getting more and more activated and energized using just one technique, one of *many* tools in her toolbox available to her!

Energizing Imagery

Energizing Imagery is a proven technique commonly used by endurance athletes. When lactic acid builds up in the muscles of athletes participating in endurance sports, athletes will experience pain and fatigue, and rely on strategies to "break through" that period and keep going. Energizing Imagery is one of the several techniques that may be leveraged (Burton and Raedeke, 2008). As human beings, we are very imaginative. The images we can create are endless, from a well-oiled high-performance Italian sports car, to a powerful animal such as Lucy's cheetah, to a powerful locomotive. You can even imagine the water you drink from your water bottle as an "energy booster" if needed. Or, once you finish tying your sneakers, imagine you have just started up your "energy shoes" (Burton and Raedeke, 2008). Endurance athlete or not, Energizing Imagery is a powerful techniques for *all* of us on our journey of health behavior change. Try it for yourself!

Self-Talk or Psyching Up

A growing body of evidence exists to support the use of positive self-talk or "psyching up" techniques in activating and sustaining positive results for health behavior change. As a psychological method for improving self-confidence, self-talk must be positive, not negative, in both our thoughts *and* words. We know that Automatic Thoughts affect our moods and confidence, and how to redirect negative thoughts to positive ones as a way to improve arousal, our moods, self-confidence, and resulting health behaviors (Chapter 5). Self-talk is most effective when it is brief, simple, effective, and relevant to you and your situation (Cox, 2012). Let's look at how the three primary types of self-talk in the form of cue words, phrases, or sentences may be used to improve our self-efficacy to change health behavior.

Three Primary Types of Self-Talk

1. **Task-Specific:** Task-specific self-talk is specific to the task needed to be accomplished. Jon, the America's Cup crew grinder, used task-specific self-talk when he exclaimed,

"Haul it up!" Someone who may be seeking to improve stress levels may tell him- or herself, "Take five and breathe!" Someone else working on controlling portion size may tell him- or herself when to "push away" (from the kitchen table) or "enough!"

2. **Encouragement of Effort:** Encouragement of effort provides just that: encouragement to push harder, keep going in the face of adversity, or set a pace. Encouragement of effort self-talk can be used with all types of behavior change. Examples include, "I am strong and I am not giving up!"; "I am committed to this and I am sticking to it!"; "Tomorrow is another day; things will get better!"; and "I've got more in me; push harder."

3. **Mood:** Finally, self-talk can affect our moods, increasing or decreasing arousal or temptation to engage in a problem behavior. For example, if you are trying to quit drinking alcohol and find yourself at an event where others were drinking, and you experience urges to drink, examples of self-talk could be "I can get through this!" or "I have come too far! I won't give in!"

Positive Affirmations

Positive affirmations are another form of self-talk. At one time or another, many of us may have experienced some kind of inner dialogue going on in our minds. Unfortunately, most inner dialogue is negative. In fact, it has been noted that up to 90 percent of self-talk is negative (Masuda, Hayes, Sackett, and Twohig, 2004)! Positive affirmations, as thoughts or words, help combat negative internal dialogue. The goal is to replace negative self-talk with positive self-talk or inner dialogue. Positive affirmations are most effective when spoken out loud. You can look in the mirror and repeat the most effective ones for you throughout the day for reinforcement and encouragement. Inspire yourself with your positive affirmations, replace mental negativity with positivity, change negative Core Beliefs, and increase your self-efficacy to maximize personal success. Change your mind, change your health! Examples of positive affirmations include:

- "I am strong."
- "I am capable."
- "I am committed."
- "I am empowered!"
- "I will keep calm and carry on today."
- "I will achieve my daily goals today."
- "I can successfully self-change."
- "I got this!" (My favorite!)
- "Let's do this!" (Another one of my favorites!)
- Or a line from a song that inspires you, such as "I am a champion, and you're gonna hear me roar!" (from Katy Perry's "Roar")

Journal Activity

List some of your positive affirmations.

Key Points

- Intrinsic Motivation is critical to sustain permanent behavior change.
- There are three dimensions of intrinsic motivation:
  - Motivation toward knowledge.
  - Motivation toward achievement.
  - Motivation toward experiencing stimulation.
- Mental Practice, also known as imagery, mental rehearsal, or visualization, is a proven effective strategy in health behavior change.
- Energizing Imagery can increase motivation for behavior change.
- Self-talk and positive affirmations are effective strategies to initiate *behavior change*, and to energize and improve *maintenance* of behavior change.

Action Items

- Use your journal to reflect, identify, and document:
  - How your SMART goals relate to the three dimensions of intrinsic motivation.
  - Mental practice ideas.
  - Suggestions for Energizing Imagery.
  - Self-talk and positive affirmations.

Part II
Sustaining Change

8

Pushing Through Lifecycle Events

Keys to Sustaining Change
Through Challenging Events

As previously mentioned, one of the most painful experiences of my life was going through my late husband Mark's brave battle with leukemia for nearly two years. The sadness, anxiety, and stress of this lifecycle event triggered my emotional eating habits, poor sleep habits, and physical inactivity. I was in the middle of a tough battle for my husband's life, caring for our 3-year-old son, our business, and our home. I spent the last year of Mark's life running back and forth to the oncology unit of the Brigham and Women's Hospital in Boston, Massachusetts, more than 100 miles away from home, trying to cope with my "new normal," until Mark sadly passed away. I was devastated. I suddenly became a widow and single mother at 33 years of age. Mark was just 36 years old. He was a healthy triathlete who did everything right to maintain his health. This was one of the reasons I found myself resenting the fact he got ill. *Why* Mark? He took such good care of himself! I spent the first four months after Mark's funeral thinking to myself, "How does a healthy lifestyle matter?"

However, I lost sight of the fact that it was because of Mark's excellent health, and his lifestyle habits, that he qualified for an aggressive, experimental leukemia treatment protocol. He had a high probability of *complete* cure. As a result of his excellent baseline health status, he was able to recover quicker from each aggressive round of treatment over the course of 18 months. Mark's leukemia was, indeed, cured! Mark's actual cause of death was pneumonia brought on from a weakened immune system resulting from the aggressive rounds of chemotherapy and radiation treatments and a bone marrow transplant. After 18 months of enduring all of the side effects of treatment, Mark, although cancer-free, was not able to respond to the antibiotic treatment for his pneumonia. Although the treatment was successful, Mark still sadly passed away. I will always admire Mark's "mental toughness," perseverance, and true grit to beat cancer!

Prior to Mark's illness, I was extremely fit and took great care of myself. After his death, I began to ignore my health. I felt physically as well as mentally horrible. I was so exhausted. I couldn't even think of exercising, and I was literally numb. When I was faced with food choices that I previously would make good and conscious decisions about, now I would simply say to myself, "Who cares?"; "I deserve to have another piece of cake."; "My world is falling apart!" However, because of spending most of my life in the health and wellness field, I intuitively knew that my poor eating habits and physical inactivity were only making my situation worse. I knew the root causes of my problem health behaviors were extreme grief and stress that manifested as a lack of motivation and commitment to my health. It was only after I began to accept and cope with the lifecycle event of Mark's death that I was able to keep my previous healthy lifestyle from totally spiraling out of control.

When I stopped justifying my poor choices with excuses for my behavior, I began to learn how to manage, as best I could, with my new "normal." I had to start to re-create a healthy lifestyle to be compatible with my changed life, now full of fears and additional responsibilities.

What Are Lifecycle Events?

Have you ever used a type of exercise equipment that had a "random intensity" programming feature? This feature, found on many types of exercise equipment such as a stationary bicycle or treadmill, randomly intensifies a workout session without a pattern or warning. The intensity may vary on a scale from one to 10. Sometimes you may find yourself at intensity level three, sometimes at intensity level 10. This is what lifecycle events are like. I define lifecycle events as events that occur in your life that are not necessarily based on your stage of life, but life events themselves. Often, they may be independent of each other. One may not know when lifecycle events will occur, and the frequencies and intensities at which they do occur may vary greatly.

We cannot predict what lifecycle events we may face during the course of our lives, when we may face them, how well positioned (or not) we will be to face them, or the impact that they will have on our lives or the lives of others. We may not know if we will face them alone or have adequate social and financial support to help us get through. Lifecycle events, often unexpected, may occur at the most inopportune times of our lives, and can be positive *or* negative.

Death of a loved one, divorce, diagnosis of a life-threatening disease, family illness, personal conflicts, financial hardship, going away to college, getting married, losing a job, starting a new job, work conflicts, coping with the aftermath of natural disasters, and having a baby are all examples of lifecycle events. Positive *or* negative lifecycle events can affect the positive health behavior changes we have made in our lives. The experience of a significant change or simultaneous changes in our lives may derail us from our journey toward positive behavior change, unless we make a conscious effort to identify changes in our behavior early and make a plan to manage them.

For those of you who may be feeling stressed or depressed, or feeling the weight of your current life situation or lifecycle event, and struggling with attaining or maintaining positive health behaviors, you are not alone. Many people must cope with all types of difficulties that affect their lifestyle behaviors. Remember: You don't have to cope alone, and don't hesitate to seek professional help when needed. Lifecycle events can sometimes make one feel hopeless and demoralized regarding sustaining positive health behavior change. Changing your mind and changing your health encourage you to seek the support you need, and allow you to slow down or "hit pause" during challenging lifecycle events. They also provide the strategies and techniques to keep pushing toward change so as not to get stuck in or resume previous health behaviors that were once mastered.

Early Detection: Increasing Awareness About Lifecycle Events

In the spring of 2010, Rhode Island experienced three days of record-breaking rain resulting in severe flooding that damaged or destroyed homes, businesses, schools, savings, and livelihoods. On the morning of March 31, 2010, the Pawtuxet River, a main river flowing to and from the Scituate Reservoir, the largest body of freshwater in the state, crested at 21 feet. This caused the worst flooding in more than 200 years for the area and forced evacuations across Rhode Island and southeastern Massachusetts.

Jill, a single professional, lived on the Pawtuxet River for eight years before her home was destroyed by the flood. She had invested most of her life savings and took out a significant amount of additional money through a home-improvement loan even before the flood struck. Jill had installed an above-ground sand filtration septic system due to the regulatory requirements of living so close to the state reservoir, waterproofed her basement, installed a new furnace, and made other needed upgrades and improvements. Just six months after these investments and improvements, the floods came without warning and water filled her home. Her home insurance would not cover the costs from flood damage, and her home was not considered to be in a flood zone at the time so she had no flood insurance. Even then, Jill was told that flood insurance would not cover damage from "ground water" that destroyed her home! As a result of this lifecycle event, Jill, a single professional woman, who tried to "do all the right things in life," faces emotional and increased financial hardship to this day.

As soon as this event happened, Jill told me she was aware that this event may take a toll on her health. By increasing her awareness of how this event may impact her health habits early, Jill was successful at pushing through the event by maintaining her health. Jill allowed herself days to put her health behavior change mission and goals on pause, but most days she did just enough of what she had to do to maintain her health while she retained legal representation (more debt) and tried to dig herself out of this very unfortunate and unpredictable event. Jill had a dog that she continued to walk twice a day for 30 minutes each time, but had to put all additional time for physical activity on hold to deal with the daunting amount of paperwork and phone calls related to settling on the damages to her home after a full day's work at the office. For the most part, she continued to eat well, get enough sleep, and keep up with her regular medical appointments. Slowly but surely, Jill was able to short-sale her house, find an affordable apartment, and return to her behavior change goals without a huge setback. She tried to take care of herself, to the best of her ability, through two very difficult years. When we are at our lowest points or most challenging times in life, it may very hard to be motivated to do anything, never mind practicing relaxation, being physically active, eating healthy, or getting adequate sleep. However, these may be the very things that give us the energy and stamina needed to push successfully through these events.

If one has the luxury of preparing for lifecycle events early, he or she may be able to improve self-consciousness or an acute sense of self-awareness of what is about to come. This can help with seamless and flexible adaptation of one's health goals and overall plan for health and well-being in the face of adversity. Increased consciousness and self-awareness is the first step toward any behavior change. The ability to know when lifecycle events are on the horizon is invaluable when trying to prepare for any personal challenges to maintaining positive health behavior change while going through them.

Throughout all my lifecycle events, and there have been many, I was well aware of them. However, during my first few traumatic lifecycle events, I did not stop for a minute to consider their repercussions on my health and well-being. As is the case with many people, the most challenging lifecycle events were the ones I was blindsided by. Therefore, I was not prepared to make necessary adjustments earlier, so my health and well-being suffered more than if I knew what was "coming down the road." Unless we are accurate fortune-tellers, we can only prepare and adjust our health goals and plans the best we can with the awareness that we have.

Holmes-Rahe Stress Inventory

The Holmes-Rahe Stress Inventory (1967) can be a very helpful tool to increase awareness of the stress toll from lifecycle events. This tool is effective in not only identifying at-risk events, but it rates the intensity of each event as well. This tool may help us identify and increase our awareness of extreme distress or disruption of our normal lives. As previously mentioned, lifecycle events may be positive *or* negative. They may consist of what I refer to as the "good and the great" or the "bad and the ugly" times in our lives. This scale helps us gauge the effect of the stress on our lives so we can prevent putting our health at risk and minimize negative consequences.

The Holmes-Rahe Life Stress Inventory
The Social Readjustment Rating Scale

Instructions: Mark down the point value of each of these life events that has happened to you during the previous year. Total the associated points.

Life Event	Mean Value
Death of spouse	100
Divorce	73
Martial separation from mate	65
Detention in jail or other institution	63
Death of a close family member	63
Major personal injury or illness	53
Marriage	50
Being fired at work	47
Marital reconciliation with mate	45
Retirement from work	45
Major change in the health or behavior of a family member	44
Pregnancy	40
Sexual difficulties	39

Gaining a new family member (i.e., birth, adoption, older adult moving in, etc.)	39
Major business readjustment	39
Major change in financial state (i.e., a lot worse or better off than usual)	38
Death of a close friend	37
Changing to a different line of work	36
Change in the number of arguments w/spouse (a lot more or less than usual regarding child rearing, personal habit, etc.)	35
Taking on a mortgage (for home, business, etc.)	31
Foreclosure on a mortgage or loan	30
Major change in responsibilities at work (i.e., promotion, demotion, etc.)	29
Son or daughter leaving home (marriage, attending college, joined military.)	29
In-law troubles	29
Outstanding personal achievement	28
Spouse beginning or ceasing work outside the home	26
Beginning or ceasing formal schooling	26
Major change in living condition (new home, remodeling, deterioration of neighborhood or home, etc.)	25
Revision of personal habits (dress manners, associations, quitting smoking)	24

Troubles with the boss	23
Major changes in working hours or conditions	20
Changes in residence	20
Changing to a new school	20
Major change in usual type and/or amount of recreation	19
Major change in church activity (i.e., a lot more or less than usual)	19
Major change in social activities (clubs, movies, visiting, etc.)	18
Taking on a loan (car, tv, freezer, etc)	17
Major change in sleeping habits (a lot more or a lot less than usual)	16
Major change in number of family get-togethers	15
Major change in eating habits (a lot more or less food intake, or very different meal hours or surroundings)	15
Vacation	13
Major holidays	12
Minor violations of the law (traffic tickets, jaywalking, disturbing the peace, etc.)	11

Now, add up all the points you have to find your score.

- **150 points or less** means a relatively low amount of life change and a low susceptibility to stress-induced health breakdown.

- 🐾 **150 to 300 points** implies about a 50 percent chance of a major health breakdown in the next two years.
- 🐾 **300 points or more** raises the odds to about 80 percent, according to the Holmes-Rahe statistical prediction model.

The Good, the Great, the Bad, and the Ugly

"Life is like a box of chocolates. You never know what you're gonna get."
—Forrest Gump

At one time or another, all of us will encounter stressful lifecycle events, whether "the good and the great" or the "bad and the ugly." And sometimes they can be both, which I describe as the "Combo Plate." All of these events—the good, the great, the bad, and the ugly can result in a very intense "overload" on normal daily life and bring on negative health consequences if they are not effectively managed. Even the good and great events can take their toll. Acute awareness of all these types of lifecycle events can help us prepare for and adapt to the sometimes-random chutes and ladders of life.

The Bad and the Ugly!

We all have our stories of the bad and ugly. I will give you snapshots of the ones that I have experienced in my life to date. At the age of 23, I experienced the tragic sudden loss of my beloved brother, Dino. He was only 19 years old. Dino was much too young to leave our family and this world! He was a kind and gentle soul. Thirty years later, his death still brings tears to my eyes, and a part of my heart will always be broken due to the loss of my dear, sweet brother. As previously mentioned, just 10 years later, at the age of 33, I lost my husband, Mark. Although some said it was expected, it was also sudden due to the fact that he was cancer-free after his treatment. I lost my husband while my 3-year-old son lost his father. At 33 years of age, I became a widow and a single mother overnight. I simply could not understand how this could happen, even to this very day. Losses of loved ones did not end here.

Seven years after Mark's death, my Portuguese grandparents (vovô and vovó) passed. I loved them dearly. It was a huge loss, as they were like second parents to me. I miss their words of wisdom, support, and love every day. In 2005, my father, my "rock," my protector, the man who always knew the right thing to say, or not say, to make me feel better, and who was always there for me to lean on, passed. The sting of his passing lingers nine years later, to this day. And, most recently, my mother was diagnosed with an early-stage, but aggressive type of breast cancer. She has endured multiple surgeries, chemotherapy, radiation, and all the side effects. I thank God that her prognosis is good, as her breast cancer was detected early through an annual mammogram. Nevertheless, it has and continues to be a difficult journey.

Sometimes I feel the grief has just piled on over the years. Through many of these events, I felt myself spiraling down while, at the same time, watching like a bystander. As those of you know who have experienced difficult lifecycle events, especially in waves, they can seem surreal, and they can take their cumulative toll on our health and well-being if we let them. Sometimes, I was able to sustain my positive health changes; sometimes I was not. However, each of these experiences increased my awareness and ability to face the next challenge with greater self-efficacy, and more rapidly recognize solutions and implement strategies to sustain my health. My personal losses have also helped me become more compassionate and understanding of others who have gone through or will go through similar events. In addition, they have given me a panoramic view of the many hills and valleys of life that we all face.

Today, as I routinely take my mother for her cancer treatments and follow-up visits at the hospital, I am mindful of others who are also living day-to-day with the long-term pressure and stress of personal or family illness. In waiting rooms, I see family members caring for their disabled children while trying to ensure their other loved ones also receive the medical treatment and care they need. You or someone dear to you may be in the middle of a high-intensity lifecycle event. You may be one of those individuals trying to "do it all" while simultaneously trying to manage the many daily details and demands of life. You are not alone, as this is a stark reality for many. I challenge you to employ the techniques presented in this chapter during your darkest *and* brightest lifecycle events, making note that caregivers sometimes need the most support, as the following quote underscores:

> *"Put yourself first. You can't be anything for anybody else unless you take care of yourself."*
> —Unknown

All of our lifecycle events place us somewhere along the Holmes-Rahe stress scale. By using this scale and gauging the impact these events had, have, or will have, on our health and well-being, we will be more enabled to develop and implement a successful sustainability plan for positive health behavior change. The mission and goal of this book are to help inspire and sustain change throughout *all* the frequencies, intensities, and times of our lives, including lifecycle events. It *is* possible for each and every one of us to accomplish!

The Good and the Great!

With the bad and ugly come the good and great, and I have been blessed to know both. In 1985, at 25 years of age, I married my first love, Mark Connolly. In our first year of marriage, we purchased our own small business (a health club) and home together, quite an achievement for us both! Five years later, we were blessed with the "sunshine of our lives," Kyle. What a lifelong, enriching experience the miracle of a child can bring! After Mark passed and I sold our business, God gave me the strength to return to school to complete my master's degree in the psycho-social aspects of Kinesiology, and I was given a valuable opportunity to conduct research on a variety of projects related to exercise physiology and the psychosocial aspects of behavior change at the University of Rhode Island. Six years after Mark's passing, I met a wonderful, honorable man of strong character, my best friend to this day, Greg Belanger. On a blistery cold winter's day, he came into a coffee shop in town while I was reading a stack of research articles, trying to figure out what the heck I was reading. We had seen each other around town many times before, so we struck up a conversation. Who knew I would get a second chance at love? Today, I have been able to watch my son grow up to be a talented artist and a kind, caring young man. I have an enjoyable and rewarding career in health and wellness that provides me with purpose, and I am publishing this, my second book, on health behavior change within four years. In the darkness, it is hard to see the light, but the sun does rise.

The Combo Plate

Sometimes we may experience a combination of different lifecycle events that put a lot on our "plate" simultaneously, while maximizing the intensity of their effect on our health. This Combo Plate may include the good, the bad, the great, *and* the ugly. For example, within weeks of being notified that Career Press/New Page Books wanted me to submit this book, my mother was diagnosed with breast cancer. So, for the past six months, I have been holding a Combo Plate of both the great and ugly. Elation over the opportunity to write this book to share my experiences and insights into achieving and sustaining personal health and well-being came with the demands of caregiving and the worry, stress, and fear about my mother's health. On a daily basis, I do my best to juggle the demands of caring for my mother and family, my professional work, and writing this book. Many of us, at various points in our lives, are challenged with juggling multiple balls in the air, while trying to maintain some type of balance between our health and life's continual demands.

Journal Activity

Make a list of the good (and great) and bad (and ugly) lifecycle events you have experienced.

Ask yourself:

- ❧ How have I sustained or maintained my health through these events?
- ❧ Did I sustain my health differently during the good versus bad events?
- ❧ How will I approach sustaining my health if faced with similar events now and in the future?

Which Path Will You Choose?

Throughout the course of 30 years in the health and wellness industry, I have personally experienced and observed others typically choosing one of the following two possible paths during lifecycle events:

1. Pushing toward change or *maintaining* positive health behaviors in spite of the challenges posed by lifecycle events (the optimal path).

2. Slowing down the pace of *action* while achieving or *maintaining* behavior change by "pressing pause" when needed. This path is especially common when striving for the "highest intensity" or most challenging change goals during the most challenging lifecycle events. Here a refined or redefined goal may be to *maintain* positive health behavior changes made to date and focus on stress management until one has the ability to resume steps toward achieving higher intensity or additional goals for behavior change.

We do not need to react to challenging lifecycle events by backsliding on the positive health behavior change(s) we have made.

Pushing Toward Change

Sometimes we are faced with the need to adjust or re-create our lifestyles as a result of lifecycle events. When my late husband, Mark, was in the hospital in Boston for weeks at a time, I would often spend entire days with him. Frequently I *contemplated* going outside for a walk, but my time with him was precious and my energy was lacking from the stress of the ordeal. At our health club, I taught multiple exercise classes per week and worked out with weights, but it was more than 100 miles away from the hospital, so I didn't have access to my normal routine. Even if I did, I didn't have the stamina to return to the club to work out once I was home, with all the running around, stress, and (single) parenting responsibilities. So, working out at the health club was not an option for me during this time. I was not accustomed to walking or running as a substitute for my traditional exercise classes and weights. However, I accepted the fact that I needed to adapt to my current situation or lifecycle event if I was going to maintain my physical *and* emotional health. The "routine" that allowed me to maintain my positive health behaviors was simply not available to me during this time in my life. I had two choices: adapt or spiral down the continuum of change.

One day, Mark's oncologist ordered a series of tests that required him to be out of his hospital room for a few hours. On that day I decided to go outside and go to a park that I drove by every day on my way to the hospital. It was in walking distance and had a walking path around a pond. Although I didn't have my sneakers with me, I went for a one-hour walk anyway. Just the sensory experience of being outside the hospital in fresh air on that beautiful summer day produced an immediate positive mental and physical response. The fragrance and sight of the flowers and trees in bloom, the soft breeze and sunlight upon my face, and the sound and laughter of children playing all lifted my spirits. *Life presented itself* to me just by being outdoors, a stark contrast to many hours spent in the somber environment of an oncology unit of a hospital. Those of you who have spent weeks, months, or even years in acute or long-term care medical settings know the grief of personal physical and emotional pain, or the grief of witnessing the suffering of others. The day that I stepped out of that environment, even for just an hour, was very healing to my being. I was in the *termination* stage of health behavior change for decades prior to that event (Chapter 1). Making the simple adaptation of going for a walk in a nearby park, which I continued to do throughout the rest of Mark's days in the hospital, helped me and my family immensely. It helped me emotionally, as well as physically continue to push toward change. Whether we choose to push toward change, or simply slow down the pace by "pressing pause," Returning to Recess, or implementing other strategies to support our health and well-being during challenging lifecycle events, we are not losing track of the ground we have gained on our journey of change.

Slow Down the Pace: Little Things Do Mean a Lot

Kate, a client of mine, was experiencing multiple "bad and ugly" lifecycle events and felt like she was being pushed to her limits. She was doing everything she could to hold it all together. We discussed options for her to continue to keep striving toward positive health behavior change while getting through this very intense time in her life. Kate decided the best she could do during this time was to commit to doing little things daily, when she could, until she was able to resume her full commitment to change. Because stress reduction was the Kate's primary health focus at this time, she committed to doing such things as practicing mindfulness and deep breathing techniques (Chapter 5). She also committed to park her car farther away when she went to the store or to her doctor's appointments; to eat at least one piece of fruit a day; to practice meditation daily; and to read excerpts from a book on relaxation. Kate was successfully able to accomplish these smaller health behavior goals, which did, indeed, help propel her through multiple, simultaneous lifecycle events and keep her overall health and well-being in balance.

Tips for Little Things or Small Steps Toward Change

- Eat an apple a day.
- Practice deep breathing.
- Take the stairs instead of the elevator.
- Park the car farther away from your walking destination.
- Reduce or eliminate caffeine intake.
- Get adequate sleep.
- Schedule a short, daily, pleasant activity or break for yourself.
- Return to Recess, even if just for five minutes per day.
- Call a friend for social support.
- Read an excerpt from spiritual literature (for example, the Bible) or a motivational book.

Strengthen Resilience to Sustain

Resilience is the ability to adapt well in the face of adversity, setbacks, tragedies, trauma, or significant stressful events (American Psychological Association, 2004). It is a crucial trait for effectively getting through lifecycle events and pushing toward change. Simply put, resilience is the ability to "bounce back." Resilience is based on keeping a positive outlook, happiness, and overall emotional health. It helps individuals deal with adversity in a positive way. In order to increase resilience, the goal is to focus on the positive, the good, and the great, versus the bad and the ugly. Practicing optimism as well as gratitude in our daily lives helps build resilience. Resilience is a trait that has been shown to improve with happiness (Chapter 9).

Coping Skills and Techniques

If you are experiencing a lifecycle event, and have made efforts to practice the techniques and tools presented in this book, but still struggle to achieve or even strive toward your health goals, give yourself permission to "press pause." Avoid Thinking Errors, such as all-or-nothing thinking, that may derail your goals completely (Chapter 5). To stay on a steady course, regardless of the pace, we must continually remind ourselves of our personal commitment to making positive health behavior change. If we adhere to our commitments, we can adjust our "sails" or goals, as needed, on our journeys.

Scheduling Pleasant Activities

Engagement in pleasant activities has shown to improve mood and help sustain healthy behaviors (Hobbis and Sutton, 2005).

Journal Activity

Schedule pleasant activities on your calendar for the next seven days. They need not be longer than 10 minutes. Examples may include taking a walk, eating dinner by candlelight, taking a bubble bath, reading a coffee table book, looking at a special picture book, or sitting down and enjoying one of your favorite hot or cold teas in a special cup or mug.

Something Bigger Than Me

In 1992, when Mark was struggling to survive pneumonia, I remember calling my long-time friend Donna from a hospital payphone on many occasions. Donna would read and recommend biblical Psalms to me. Along with daily prayer and the Serenity Prayer these Psalms became a source of refuge for me during some of the darkest moments of my life. Now, they are part of my nighttime ritual. I also repeat an old adage that has helped sustain me through many difficult times: "This too shall pass." No matter what one's religious beliefs are or aren't, prayer and finding a source of strength from something or someone bigger than ourselves can bring true and real strength to us in our darkest hours. A spiritual connection with a higher power has been shown to be very healing on an emotional, spiritual, as well as physical level (Aten, O'Grady, and Worthington, 2011).

Once I was privileged to spend an afternoon with Dan Buettner, an internationally recognized researcher, explorer, *New York Times* best-selling author, and National Geographic Fellow. Dan founded Blue Zones®, a company that puts the world's best practices in longevity and well-being to work in people's lives. Dan has traveled the world, researching common threads of people who and communities that live the longest. What he has found he shares in one of his best-selling books, *The Blue Zones: Lessons for Living Longer From the People Who've Lived the Longest* (2010). Dan states that one of the nine keys to living a long, healthy, and happy life is a sense of belonging and being part of a faith-based organization. Dan's research shows that attending faith-based services, no matter what denomination, at least four times per month can add up to 14 years to one's life expectancy! Dan's research demonstrates that regular participation in a faith-based community and the belief in something bigger than ourselves improve both well-being and longevity.

Practicing Gratitude

Martin Seligman, author of *Flourish* (2011), found that gratitude can add to life satisfaction and personal happiness. When practicing gratitude, we can benefit from recalling pleasant events that have added meaning and purpose to our lives or in some way changed our lives for the better. If we do not intentionally spend time practicing gratitude, it may be easy to forget these events over time. Seligman also found that when we express gratitude toward others, we strengthen our relationships with them, which, in turn, enriches our lives and builds stronger social supports. In *Flourish*, Seligman suggests an exercise called "The Gratitude Visit." The Gratitude Visit begins with writing a very detailed letter to someone who has positively impacted your life. It is taking the time to express your gratitude in a purposeful, meaningful way, not just with passing thoughts, but with real refection and recollection.

Like the "good and great" lifecycle event, writing a gratitude list helps us take note of all the positive events and important individuals in our lives, even in the midst of the "bad and ugly" lifecycle events. These types of exercises can help us put our lives in perspective and shine the light on the positive aspects during dark or stressful times.

Journal Activity

Ask yourself:

- ✦ Do I *always* say thank you, even for the little things?
- ✦ Do I stop and count my blessings?

If you answered yes to both questions, and do them on a regular basis, you are practicing gratitude. If not, on a daily basis, intentionally try to keep mental notes as well as an ongoing written list of all of the things, big and small, that you are grateful for. With practice we can all cultivate an "attitude of gratitude" to help us push toward change during our darkest and most difficult times.

Journal Activity

- ✦ Write your gratitude list. (Set aside 10 minutes every night before bed.)
- ✦ List three things that went well today.
- ✦ Describe the reason(s) these things went well. (For example, a stranger helped me fix my flat tire today so I was able to get to work on time.)

Key Points

- ✦ Lifecycle events are intense, predictable, *or* unpredictable events that occur throughout our life stages.
- ✦ Increasing awareness of and early detection of lifecycle events is critical to sustaining positive health behavior change throughout them.

Action Items

- ๏ Complete the Holmes-Rahe Stress Inventory.
- ๏ Make a list of your good (and great) and bad (and ugly) life-cycle events.
- ๏ Complete Journal Activities.
- ๏ Schedule pleasant activities.
- ๏ Keep a daily gratitude list.

9

Ways to Well-Being

Happiness Can Change Your Mind,
Change Your Health!

My late Portuguese grandfather (Avô), Eduino, my mother's father, was a happy and wise man with a wonderful and positive outlook on life. To this day, he is an inspiration to my personal well-being. Avô had a deep appreciation and love for life, his family, and nature. Every day, he basked in the simple things, rain or shine, from sunrise to sunset. He marveled at all of life's beauty. Avô always counted his blessings and was an optimistic person who held hope and a glass always half-full. As many before and after him, he came to America by boat from the one of the nine Azorean islands of Portugal, Faial, from the city of Horta, to Ellis Island in 1920. He came at the young age of 15 accompanied by his sister, Olivia (Olive), who was pregnant at the time. I can't imagine how scared he must have been, leaving his country and parents at such a young age while being responsible for Olive. But, he had hope and a *vision*, and he achieved his goals! When he arrived in the United States, he stayed with family and was given an opportunity to work as a shoemaker's apprentice. During and after the Great Depression, shoe repair or cobbling was a relatively profitable trade compared to others, as people could not afford to purchase new shoes.

Around 1930, Avô met and soon married the love of his life, my grandmother (*Avóa*). In 1940, he opened his own shoe store and repair shop, The Town Shoe Store, in East Providence, Rhode Island. Avô went on to purchase his own home and start a family. He continued to persevere very hard at his trade, eventually saving enough money to build his own building in the early 1950s as he continued to operate and grow a successful business. In addition to shoe sales and repair, my Avô served as a building manager for several other small businesses that rented space in his building.

Avô was a self-educated man dedicated to continual learning and self-improvement throughout his life. During his youth in Portugal, he performed in the theater, which he continued to do after immigrating to the United States. A vibrant member of the Portuguese-American community, Avô performed in numerous Portuguese plays in the southern New England area. He loved literature and poetry, and learned to recite Shakespeare in English, his second language.

Our close-knit, extended Portuguese family spent a lot of time at my grandparents' home, the gathering hub for relatives and close friends. Avô planted fruit trees in his yard and had a garden in the back of his shoe store where he grew a variety fresh fruits and vegetables. *Avóa* (my grandmother), an excellent cook, prepared balanced, healthy meals with fresh ingredients from their beautiful garden. They generously shared their home and meals with family members, friends, and neighbors on a daily basis. At a time where "cleaning your plate" was the norm, for Avô, practicing moderation was a key part of his lifestyle. He would often say, *"Always leave the table knowing you could eat a little more."* Avô wasn't a big drinker, but had an occasional glass of red wine with dinner, and would remedy a "tickle" in his throat in the cold months with an occasional small shot of whiskey. He practiced a healthy, balanced lifestyle long before the concept of well-being emerged. Avô loved to sing and he would always remind me when I went home for my frequent visits to "keep singing." He loved watching cartoons and old Charlie Chaplin silent movies. When we joined him for breakfast at the local restaurant, Avô would often draw figures of Charlie on napkins for my son, Kyle (then a toddler), to keep him entertained.

He aged gracefully and maintained his sense of humor. I fondly remember his April Fool's Day practical jokes and other pranks. One Halloween evening, when I was a teenager, Avô grabbed and climbed up a ladder that my father kept around the back of our house for painting. Avô used the ladder to climb two stories high after adorning himself with a horrifying mask and black cape. As my mother approached the sink to do the evening dishes, she saw him through the window in the dark shadows of the night! My mother screeched for all the neighbors to hear. My brother, father, uncle, grandmother, and I all giggled and laughed about it for years!

My Avô was a respected, prominent, and active member of the local business and church community. In addition, he founded the Portuguese Cultural Association, whose mission was to educate first- and second-generation Portuguese children on the importance of their culture in order to provide a voice for the future of the Portuguese community in the state of Rhode Island. He received awards and recognition for his seemingly endless contributions and dedication to the Portuguese Cultural Association. Avô would often practice acts of kindness among the people in his community. For example, he repaired the shoes of the poor and the church leaders at no charge. Avô had a strong faith and was actively involved in his church.

My grandparents walked everywhere. East Providence, like many towns before the Second World War, was of typical "street grid" design, with traditional, mix-used neighborhoods. Everything one needed, including the local market and drugstore, was within walking distance. My grandparents did not even own a car until my parents and I moved from the house next door to another area of East Providence. Avô was more than 60 years old when he purchased his first car, a brand-new 1963 sky blue Ford Fairlane.

In addition to walking everywhere, Avô was very physically active. My mother speaks of her father in his 30s and 40s when she would come down the stairs to see him doing headstands and calisthenics in the living room every morning. He was an outdoorsman who enjoyed nature and fishing. He kept himself physically fit and at a healthy body weight for most of his long life.

Avô was not one to harbor resentments or bitterness. He remained physically and mentally healthy throughout his long life, and aged with peace and grace. To this day, we say my grandfather died of a broken heart after his bride of 68 years passed less than a year before him. Avô passed without any chronic health conditions at 95. He fulfilled his American dream and lived a life full of love, meaning, hard work, and passion.

Unbeknownst to me at the time, my grandfather's life was a story of true well-being, perseverance, and personal achievement. In this chapter, we will explore the theory of positive psychology and well-being and how it may be applied to support and sustain behavior change.

Journal Activity

- List the people in your life who exhibit some of the positive characteristics of happiness, optimism, perseverance, humor, positive relationships, and active engagement in life.
- List the people in your life who practice acts of kindness.
- Talk to these individuals and ask them about their outlook on life.
- Take notes how you can model their behaviors.
- Seek opportunities to learn from them through Vicarious Experiences and Observational Learning (Chapter 4).

Positive Psychology: The Next Step in Our Journey of Change

Once we have achieved success on our journey of change, what's next? We must maintain our results. By continuing to utilize the assessments, strategies, and techniques in this book, termination *is* achievable. Striving toward total well-being can also assist in maintaining the positive changes to improve our health and quality of life, simply by improving or optimizing our outlook on life.

In the last decade, we have seen the growth of positive psychology, a fairly new branch of psychology. The field of psychology has shifted from mental illness to the area of positive human potential and growth, forming the basis of the positive psychology movement. Positive psychology focuses on positive affective states, such as emotions, moods, emotional traits, and sentiments. It also focuses on positive aspects of well-being to include, but not limited to, positive emotions, happiness, hope, and optimism. Positive psychology encompasses constructs of well-being, contentment, and life satisfaction (in the past); hope and optimism (for the future); and engagement, flow, and happiness (in the present) (Seligman, 2011).

Positive *emotions*, along with positive thoughts, can help us make better lifestyle choices, improve social supports, and improve our ability to cope with stress (Chapter 5). Increasing mindfulness of our thoughts and emotions can help us thrive or flourish in our lives. However, caution exists when one experiences excessive optimism, particularly if it results in a distorted belief that can work against us or cause us harm. For example, if we ignore the need to seek help due to serious health and emotional issues by not being realistic or falsely optimistic, this could be detrimental to our health. Therefore, the field of positive psychology does not recommend elimination of appropriate negative emotions. It is important to regulate both positive *and* negative emotions to ensure that there is a healthy balance between the two. An ideal ratio of three positive emotions to every one negative emotion is recommended to achieve positive emotional well-being (Algoe and Fredrickson, 2011).

Journal Activity

- ‿ Be mindful of your positive and negative emotions.
- ‿ Maintain an appropriate balance or ratio of positive and negative emotions.

Be Happy!

A large body of evidence demonstrates that people who are happier achieve better life outcomes. These outcomes can include financial success, meaningful relationships, emotional health, effective coping abilities, physical health, and longevity (Cohn, Fredrickson, Brown, Mikels, and Conway, 2009). Happiness is made up of a combination of characteristics and personality traits including life satisfaction, coping ability, positive emotions, and outlook. The bottom line is individuals that are more satisfied with their lives perform better in most, if not all, aspects of their lives. The research does not define happiness as "cheerfulness," smiling, or merriment, but rather positive life satisfaction. Happiness is about valued experiences that *we* perceive as meaningful, not experiences that others value. Happiness, a critical component of positive psychology, assists us with maintaining behavior change over time and improving our quality of life. Dr. Seligman defines happiness as a multifaceted construct that can be broken down into three subjective and distinct types of well-being. They include pleasure or positive emotions, engagement, and meaning, all three of which improve life satisfaction (Jayawickreme, Forgeard, and Seligman, 2012). Each type of well-being is described later in this chapter.

It has been proposed that happy people have greater life satisfaction not simply because they feel better, but because they developed the skills and possessed or acquired the personality traits described in this chapter, leveraged resources to improve coping skills, and achieved elements of well-being (Cohn, et al., 2009). To improve our well-being, we must evaluate and continuously make the necessary adjustments or improvements in our lives to optimize life satisfaction. Rate your life satisfaction with the following scale.

Satisfaction With Life Scale

Using the scale provided, rate your response to each of the statements below.

7 = Strongly agree

6 = Agree

5 = Slightly agree

4 = Neither agree nor disagree

3 = Slightly disagree

2 = Disagree

1 = Strongly disagree

_____ In most ways my life is close to my ideal.

_____ The conditions of my life are excellent.

_____ I am satisfied with my life.

_____ So far I have gotten the important things I want in life.

_____ If I could live my life over, I would change almost nothing.

Total Score: _____

31–35 = Extremely satisfied

26–30 = Satisfied

21–25 = Slightly satisfied

20 = Neutral

15–19 = Slightly dissatisfied

10–14 = Dissatisfied

5–9 = Extremely dissatisfied

(Adapted from Diener, Emmons, Larsen, and Griffin, 1985)

Journal Activity

- List any statements that you may have scored low on and want to improve.
- List ways that you can improve your score on these statements or your overall score.

Well-Being

The construct of happiness evolved into the theory of well-being in 2011. The theory of well-being includes but goes beyond happiness. "Well-being is also about positive virtues and traits such as capacity to love, vocation, honesty, perseverance, hope, work ethic, forgiveness, originality, future minded, spirituality, and wisdom" (Seligman and Csikszentmihalyi, 2000). In his book *Flourish*, Dr. Seligman describes the similarities among well-being and weather and freedom, in that no one single element, structure, or measure defines it completely. Well-being is subjective in nature; it is *what people think or feel about their lives*. An individual's temperament and personality appear to be powerful factors in subjective well-being, in part because individuals usually adapt to good or bad conditions to some degree (Diener, 2000).

Elements of well-being have been developed, including those by Gallup, Inc., an American research-based, global performance-management consulting company founded by George Gallup in 1935. Gallup,

Inc. is well known for its public opinion polls, conducted in the United States and other countries. Gallup's global well-being metrics and improvement systems inform strategies for tracking and transforming the health of individuals, organizations, and communities. Gallup's five interdependent elements of well-being are:

- **Career Well-Being:** Are you enriched by and satisfied with your work? If you enjoy what you do for work and look forward to going to work every day, you are twice as likely to thrive.

- **Social Well-Being:** Do you have meaningful relationships in your life? Similar to other definitions of well-being and theories of behavior change, those with strong social supports are likely to thrive.

- **Financial Well-Being:** Do you feel secure and satisfied with your financial situation? This element doesn't necessarily mean you are happy with the amount of money you have, or the amount of money you make. Financial well-being is more about how you are managing your finances and that your financial decisions lead to financial security, as well as your satisfaction with your standard of living.

- **Physical Well-Being:** This is an element that is most focused on in traditional "wellness" programs. It is important that you are taking care and practicing prevention to protect your physical health to the point that you achieve energy and vitality.

- **Community Well-Being:** Those who are thriving are involved and contribute to their community. Like my grandfather did, those who thrive in this element of well-being connect with their social groups and work on causes in their community that they are passionate about and fulfill their personal mission. (O'Reilly, 2013).

Seligman also identifies five elements of well-being, most overlapping with Gallup's. Seligman's elements of well-being may be remembered by the acronym PERMA: positive emotions, engagement, relationships, meaning, and accomplishment (Jayawickreme, Forgeard, and Seligman, 2012).

Positive Emotions

Positive emotions have been shown to predict resilience or one's ability to bounce back from setbacks and improve life satisfaction (Cohn, et al., 2009). In the "pleasant life," we choose to focus on our positive emotions. Positive emotions are cultivated by "taking time to smell the roses," enjoying pleasant activities, and striving to create moments of pleasure or comfort. Vacations, "staycations," or vacations spent at home, and mini-breaks throughout a busy day all help us experience the awe of life to its fullest each and every day. Happiness and life satisfaction are two important elements of our positive emotions. Despite any time constraints, we must take time to do the things that make us happy. On my list of things that make me happy is attending four or five concerts per year with my son, Kyle. I try my best to continue to make the time to fulfill my mission and goals, in spite of family and work responsibilities, time constraints, and lifecycle events.

Last evening, Kyle and I went to see one of our favorite bands, Paramore, of which Kyle is a longtime fan and friend. We have been attending their performances for more than nine years now, from Washington, D.C., to New York City, to Boston, to Nashville, to New Hampshire, and even to the Bahamas. Paramore's performances are electric. The energy and emotion that this band projects on stage through their lyrics and music evoke positive, palatable emotions in the audience. Attending concerts with my now-25-year-old son is such as positive emotional experience for me. It represents years of memories of us listening to music and singing together, from when Kyle was a toddler learning to talk, through his adolescent years, all the while enjoying a common love for music that we continue to share to this day.

Engagement

When I think of engagement, I immediately think of my husband, Greg, who truly engages in life. He completely immerses himself in the simple or "little" things such as watching a sunset, taking in the beauty of mountains while downhill skiing, listening to the birds outside the house in the early morning, and many other simple experiences that captivate his undistracted attention. All of his senses are engaged. It is truly amazing for me to witness, unless I am trying to get his attention. As a man in his 50s, Greg maintains a childlike absorption of wonder. Although it can be more challenging for me, I strive to be more engaged in my life. When my son and I visited Epcot Center, one of four theme parks at Walt Disney World, we went on the ride "Soarin'," a simulator ride in the "future world." The ride is like an exhilarating hang-gliding experience. The ride takes you through a variety of stunning, IMAX-quality images such as mountains, fields, oceans, and orange groves. It engages all your senses through beautiful sights, sounds, scents, wind, and other special effects. Minutes into the ride, I was completely engaged and immersed in the experience. I could not tell you what I was thinking or feeling at the time.

When we finished the ride, Kyle and I both turned to each other and I exclaimed with total elation, "That was *awesome*!" while Kyle exclaimed, "Wow, that was *crazy*!" Seligman refers to this type of experience as being engaged and in "flow." Being in "flow" is described as almost losing consciousness as one becomes so absorbed in an experience that "time stops." While working, we are engaged or completely immersed in projects when we are "in the zone." On Soarin', I most definitely was in a state of flow. I also found myself in "flow" last night dancing in "the pit" to many of Paramore's high-energy songs, including their newest hit single, "Ain't It Fun." To bolster our well-being, we must ensure we are engaged in life every day, even in the "smallest" or seemingly insignificant experiences of life!

Journal Activity

- ∾ Make a list of the experiences that put you in "flow."
- ∾ Add to the list ways that you can engage more in life!

Positive Relationships

Christopher Peterson, one of the founders of positive psychology, once stated that positive psychology is simply about *other people* (Seligman, 2011). If we think back on all of our experiences related to positive emotions, engagement, relationships, meaning, and accomplishment, they most likely all include other people. Throughout my life experiences detailed in this book, I describe the involvement of and impact on my family. I can also vividly recall days of meaningful experiences with friends and colleagues decades ago, although I remember them as if they were yesterday. For example, I remember a hot summer day more than 30 years ago. I was riding around the Narragansett Beach area in Narragansett, Rhode Island, with my friend Donna in her red "spitfire" convertible. We were laughing and feeling totally elated, like we didn't have a care in the world. That day, the "world was our oyster." I carry another fond memory of a picture-perfect summer day at Castle Hill Inn on Ocean Avenue in Newport, Rhode Island. I was with my dear friend Kathy as we sat outside watching a sailing race from Newport to England, enjoying a glass of wine, shrimp cocktail, and salads. Absorbed in the moment, we enjoyed being by the ocean, sharing each other's company and conversation, and mingling with the crowd during the race. That day, neither of us had a care in the world! We were so engaged in those unforgettable moments that at times it felt surreal.

Journal Activity

- ♥ Reflect on and write down positive experiences that have included your personal relationships.
- ♥ Think about how you can plan more experiences with your friends and family.

Meaning

Seligman (2011) describes meaning as "belonging to and serving something that you believe is bigger than the self." I previously described how my spiritual belief in "something bigger than me" brought me a sense of comfort during many times in my life (Chapter 8). My emotions could not bring me that comfort, nor could most of the elements of well-being previously described. However, my sense of meaning and my spiritual belief synergistically contributed to my well-being. Meaning contributes to well-being and is often sought after for its own purpose. For example, if you believe in and are active for a particular cause, and others disagree with your belief or involvement that you pursue anyway because of its meaning to you, you are fulfilling this element of well-being. Finally, meaning is defined and measured independent of positive emotions, engagement, relationships, and accomplishment.

One who pursues a career with personal meaning to him and her simultaneously pursues well-being. I pursue projects with my clients and writing about health and well-being topics because I believe in and I am passionate about the meaning they bring to my life and the lives of others. I believe the theories, strategies, and techniques presented in this book will help people improve the health and quality of their lives. Helping people change or improve their health *and* well-being gives meaning to my life, so I answered the *call* to write this book. As some of you may have experienced, there is an intense commitment in writing a meaningful book, thesis, or manuscript that sometimes is accompanied by a drain in creative and physical energy. Sometimes you or others may second-guess or question the meaning of such a commitment. The time and energy involved may take a toll on your social and family life as you see it through to a finished product. Several of my friends and family members have asked me, "Are you sure you want to go through this again?" And yes, there are many days I find myself asking myself the same question. But I continue this and similar projects because of the meaning and purpose it brings to my life.

Journal Activity

- Reflect on and write down what gives you meaning in your life.
- Are you pursuing these things?
- If not, how can you start to pursue meaningful things in your life?

Accomplishment

Accomplishments are most valuable when they are pursued for intrinsic versus extrinsic motivations. Accomplishments that provide meaning and purpose increase life satisfaction and well-being. Throughout my career, I have been fortunate to meet and learn from many highly accomplished individuals. Many strived for accomplishment, not for money or fame, but because they believed in what they were doing and were motivated to succeed or even excel. One of the most significant mentors, and among the admired people in my life, Dr. James O. Prochaska, who wrote the Foreword for this book, is a leading international authority in health behavior change. As a psychologist, Dr. Prochaska has pursued more than four decades of research, making worldwide contributions to the field of health behavior change by adding a significant body of evidence to support his Transtheoretical Model of Behavior change developed in 1977. He did this, not for fame or glory, or monetary gain, but for the sake of *meaning* and accomplishment in the field of behavioral psychology and to help people *thrive*.

Journal Activity

- Write down examples of people, including yourself, who have achieved a high level of accomplishment.
- What can you learn from your accomplishment and their pursuit of accomplishment?
- How can you apply what you have learned from others to your life?

Optimism

Research has demonstrated that those with a high degree of optimism, a dispositional personality trait of positive psychology, tend to have improved moods, greater perseverance in the face of adversity, are more successful, and are in better physical health (Diener, 2000). If we have an optimistic disposition, we are more likely to be able to successfully navigate unexpected or challenging external events and make more positive interpretations of them (Diener, 2000). If we are optimistic, we are more likely to achieve our health behavior goals, in spite of any life-cycle events or other barriers we may encounter on our journey of change.

There is a difference between "little" optimism and "big" optimism. An example of an expression of little optimism is "I know I will start preparing to quit smoking today by calling the quit line." An example of an expression of big optimism is "I know I will quit and quit permanently in the next year." To increase the level of optimism in your thinking patterns, begin with "little" optimistic thoughts, and gradually and intentionally try to change them to "big" optimistic thoughts. Daily practice and monitoring will help you become successful at changing your way of thinking.

Journal Activity

- ✤ Use your daily journal to track your thoughts related to how optimistic you are about challenging situations you may be facing that negatively impact your health and well-being.

- ✤ Differentiate between your little and big optimistic thoughts or reactions.

Practice Random Acts of Kindness

In his research, Seligman found that practicing acts of kindness actually produces the single-most momentary increase in well-being than any other action (Seligman, 2011). Acts of kindness can brighten both the giver's and the receiver's days. Eva was on her way home from Boston to the University of Rhode Island, and had a one-and-a-half-hour drive home. Midway there, she realized that her gas tank was on empty and that she had left her wallet at home. Arriving at the nearest gas station, Eva scraped up the change that she could find in her car, and walked in to speak with the gas station cashier. Embarrassingly, Eva lay out her change on the counter, apologizing for and explaining her dilemma. As she was literally counting out her pennies on the counter, an elderly man, wearing a gas station shirt from another gas station, pulled up in his old, beat-up car, walked in, observed Eva at the counter, and told the cashier, "Hold on, I will be right back." The elderly man ran out of the gas station, went to his car, and came back and handed the cashier a $20 bill, asking Eva which car was hers. Not quite knowing how to thank the man, Eva jokingly offered him her pennies. The response he gave was one that took her aback, "God blessed me today by giving me the opportunity to help you. Just turn around and help someone else." His smile was filled with warmth and kindness, and his eyes were shinning with wisdom. This random act of kindness that was performed out of the goodness of the man's heart, with no ulterior motive, was deeply moving and evoked strong positive emotions for both the man and Eva.

Even small acts of kindness have a positive effect on our well-being. For example, in the grocery store this week I observed a woman in front of me in the checkout line receive a bill of $20.12 for a few items that she purchased. As she riffled through the bottom of her purse for the change, as women commonly do, I happened to have my wallet out and handed her the 12 cents. At first she declined and said, "That's okay. I have it somewhere." When she was still looking, I offered again and she accepted. She was so appreciative; you would think I gave her 50 dollars! She smiled as she left the store, and, as a result of seeing her reaction, I felt like I *did* give her 50 dollars. How could such a small or minute act of kindness make me feel so good?

Acts of kindness can be small, like waiting with the door open for an elderly person, or can be larger, requiring more of our time, expertise, resources, or funding. The bottom line is kindness feels good, may boost your mood, and improves your well-being while you help someone else out in the process. It doesn't get any better than that!

Journal Activity

- ⚬ Tomorrow, find one totally unexpected kind thing you can do for someone and just do it.
- ⚬ Observe and record what happens to your mood.
- ⚬ Repeat an act or acts of kindness daily.
- ⚬ Make a list of small and large acts of kindness that you could show over the course of a week or month.

Laughter

"Laughter is the best medicine."
—Unknown

"Cheerfulness is the best promoter of health, and is as friendly to the mind as to the body."
—Joseph Addison (English essayist, poet, and dramatist, 1672–1719)

"A good laugh makes you healthy."
—Swedish Proverb

Laughter increases positive emotions (Bachorowski and Owren, 2001). Those who have a tendency to use humor as a coping skill report greater daily positive moods (Dillon, Minchoff, and Baker, 1985–1986).

Laughter, and even smiling, improves resilience in the face of adversity, loss, and trauma. Several studies of bereaved individuals found that those who experienced genuine laughs and smiles when speaking about their loss experienced better adjustment over several years of bereavement (Bonanno, 2004). Another found that higher resilience and adjustment after the September 11th attacks in New York City were influenced by the experience of positive emotions such as gratitude, interest, and love (Fredrickson, Tugade, and Larkin, 2003). President Abraham Lincoln used humor in politics to defuse tense situations and impart wisdom during some of the darkest times in American history. In the 1860s, President Lincoln prefaced a discussion of the draft for the Emancipation Proclamation by reading aloud an excerpt from a favorite humorist. In response to the disapproval of some members of his cabinet, President Lincoln said, "Gentlemen, why don't you laugh? With the fearful strain that is upon me night and day, if I did not laugh I should die, and you need this medicine as much as I do."

Journal Activity

- List ways in which you might be able to use humor and laughter to increase your positive emotions and coping abilities.

- List any comedy movies or videos of stand up comics or CDs you may enjoy that you can watch regularly to improve your mood and increase positive emotions (for example, Peter Sellers's original *Pink Panther* series of comedy films, or *Office Space,* a 1999 American comedy film written and directed by Mike Judge).

- List ways to strengthen your resilience by laughing or smiling more during "bad and ugly" lifecycle or everyday events.

Well-Being and Physical and Emotional Health

Numerous studies have linked improvements in well-being with improvements in health. One study showed that those who remained optimistic about the outcome of life-threatening diseases, such as AIDS, had delayed symptoms as well as improved survival rates compared to less optimistic patients. A consideration is that optimistic patients may practice improved health behaviors that enhance physical and emotional health, including enlisting strong social supports. Positive emotional states such as happiness and mood may also have direct physiological effects, and have been shown to slow the course of illness (Seligman and Csikszentmihalyi, 2000).

Well-being has demonstrated direct positive effects on the physiological functioning of our bodily systems, such as our immune system. However, at this time, more is known about how negative emotions promote illness than about how positive emotions promote health. The research on positive psychology has demonstrated that those who have a high degree of life satisfaction are more likely to muster up the resources and motivation to stick with positive health behaviors and goals (Seligman and Csikszentmihalyi, 2000).

Key Points

- Don't worry, be happy! People who are happier achieve better life outcomes.
- Gallup has identified five global well-being metrics and improvement systems to inform strategies for tracking and transforming the health of individuals, organizations, and communities to include:
    - Career well-being.
    - Social well-being.
    - Financial well-being.
    - Physical well-being.
    - Community well-being.
- Seligman has identified five elements of well-being (PERMA) to include:
    - Positive emotions.
    - Engagement.
    - Relationships.
    - Meaning.
    - Accomplishment.

Action Items

- ꙮ Rate your life satisfaction with the Satisfaction With Life Scale.

- ꙮ List any statements that you may have scored low on and want to improve.

- ꙮ List ways that you can improve your score on these statements or your overall score.

- ꙮ Complete Journal Activities.

- ꙮ Practice random acts of kindness.

- ꙮ Strengthen your optimism through laughter and use of humor.

10

Got Grit.

Thriving: Your Ultimate End Zone

The America's Cup Crew members possessed true grit. Most athletes, at an elite level, possess this potent virtue. Grit may be an innate trait, but athletes also train to strengthen their *grittiness*. Grit is defined as the combination of a very high perseverance and a high passion for an objective or goal (Duckworth, Peterson, Matthews, and Kelly, 2007). Both elite athletes and non-athletes may possess this extraordinary trait. Some have worked hard to learn to harness its power in setting health behavior goals and maintaining successful health behavior change. However, in the field of psychology, the question remains: "Why do most individuals make use of only a small portion of their resources, whereas a few exceptional individuals push themselves to their limits?" (Duckworth, et al., 2007) There is a large body of mounting evidence on the possession and utilization of the powerful trait of grit.

Journal Activity

Honestly answer the following two questions as they relate to your goals for behavior change and commitment (Chapter 6):

1. Are you leveraging all of your resources to maintain your successful health behavior change?
2. Are you pushing yourself to your limits to achieve your goals for behavior change?

If you answered yes to both of these questions, you have grit. If you answered no to one or both, you may increase your grittiness by leveraging all of the evidence-based resources in this book.

Strengthening Grit

The process of Self-Liberation strengthens our commitment to achieving our goals (Chapter 2). Once we have set a clear and well-defined mission and vision, and set SMART goals to achieve them, we are ready to develop a sustainability plan (Chapter 6). Using the powerful techniques from sports psychology (Chapter 7) and Cognitive Behavioral Therapy (CBT) (Chapter 5) can help improve your grittiness. When I reminisce about the thousands of people I have worked with over three decades in the health and wellness field, from academic research, to the health club industry, to public health initiatives, to corporate settings, I learned that the people who possessed and harnessed the powerful trait of grit were most likely to achieve and sustain their health behavior change over long periods of time, in spite of all obstacles and lifecycle events that could have derailed them.

Making a strong commitment (Chapter 3) and determining our mission, vision, and SMART goals (Chapter 6) are essential first steps to strengthening or building our Grit. In his book, *Flourish*, Dr. Seligman describes how his favorite social psychologist, Roy Baumeister, believes "the queen of all the virtues" is *self-discipline.* Dr. Baumeister describes self-discipline as "the strength than enables the rest of our strengths." However, Seligman's research demonstrated that grit was an even more powerful trait than self-discipline. Those who possess grit are able to successfully maintain their determination and motivation over *long* and *sustained* periods of time despite experiences with failure and adversity. When we strengthen or build our grit, we will experience the greatest success at achieving mental *and* physical behavior change for optimal health and well-being.

As my husband, Greg, says, if you look at competitive sports, usually everyone plays well in the first quarter of a game. But winners are made by how well they perform throughout the *entire* game to the end, when they may be most physically and mentally stressed, drained, and fatigued. During the 2014 FIFA World Cup hosted by Brazil, the United States played in the World Cup *elimination game* against *Belgium.* After

90 minutes of regulation time, both teams played to a zero-zero tie score. Both teams were determined in overtime play, when all players appeared physically and mentally exhausted. A sporting event like this exemplifies true grit. And, as mentioned earlier, these players train to harness this powerful virtue, and so must we, athletes or not. "It's not uncommon to hear that the winner invariably comes down to who is the strongest athlete, mentally, on a given day" (Cox, 2012). Athletics is about personal behavior change, at a competitive level, but the same concepts can be applied nonetheless. Making the original commitment to health-behavior change is much easier than maintaining that commitment over long periods of time in the face of adversity, stress, and pressure.

When I owned my health club, I was concerned about new members who were previously inactive for most of their lives. I would watch many begin working out overzealously seven days per week. Many new members, who "charged out of the gate" fast and furious, would lose momentum because they could not maintain their commitment to being physical active at such a high intensity over time. Sadly, I would watch many extremely passionate new members "fizzle out" and quit. Once I noticed this pattern, I worked with our staff to sit down with these members, compliment them on their efforts, but also offer assistance with developing a workout plan to include *gradual* increases in frequency, intensity, and duration that could be maintained over time *and* in the face of obstacles. My staff would share the anonymous stories of other new members that went full speed ahead at the onset and explain how they were unable to maintain this level of physical activity. When members saw the value in a lifelong commitment to physical activity, they were more likely to reach out to us for feedback and assistance. Our commitment to achieve our health goals is more successful when our plans are designed more in line with a "marathon" than a "sprint," and those with the most grit are those more typically able to "stay the course," for the long-haul. They have stamina to press on without detouring or derailing.

Achievement Equation

Achievement is equivalent to effort times (x) skill (Seligman, 2011). Effort is the amount of time and energy directed toward a task (such as your goals for behavior change), whereas skill is the applied knowledge we have acquired on our journey of behavior change. Knowledge of what we need to do to achieve our goals is not enough without devoting the time, energy, and effort to achieve them. Anders Ericsson, a professor at Florida State University, argues that, "The cornerstone of all high expertise is not God given genius, but deliberate practice: the amount of time and energy you spend in deliberate practice" (Seligman, 2011, p. 115). Seligman asks the question, "What determines how much time you are willing to devote to achievement?" Character and self-discipline embody deliberate practice. In order to make the substantial effort needed to achieve and maintain behavior change, we must be willing to sacrifice short-term pleasures for long-term gains. Sacrificing short-term pleasures may be very difficult, but often necessary for long-term success. Strengthening the character trait of self-discipline can help us achieve our mission and vision for health behavior change.

Got Grit.

I posed the title to this chapter as a statement, *not* as a question, because we all possess some degree of this powerful trait. However, to what degree we harness our "grit" for each of our personal goals may vary. When we learn to harness the power of grit, strengthen it, and apply it toward our goals for behavior change, we are most likely to achieve them.

Short Grit Scale

Please respond to the following eight items using the scale that follows. Be honest. There are no right or wrong answers!

1.   **New ideas and projects sometimes distract me from old ones.***
   - ☐ Very much like me
   - ☐ Mostly like me
   - ☐ Somewhat like me
   - ☐ Not much like me
   - ☐ Not like me at all

2.   **Setbacks don't discourage me.**
   - ☐ Very much like me
   - ☐ Mostly like me
   - ☐ Somewhat like me
   - ☐ Not much like me
   - ☐ Not like me at all

3. **I have been obsessed with a certain idea or project for a short time but later lost interest.***
   - ☐ Very much like me
   - ☐ Mostly like me
   - ☐ Somewhat like me
   - ☐ Not much like me
   - ☐ Not like me at all

4. **I am a hard worker.**
   - ☐ Very much like me
   - ☐ Mostly like me
   - ☐ Somewhat like me
   - ☐ Not much like me
   - ☐ Not like me at all

5. **I often set a goal but later choose to pursue a different one.***
   - ☐ Very much like me
   - ☐ Mostly like me
   - ☐ Somewhat like me
   - ☐ Not much like me
   - ☐ Not like me at all

6. **I have difficulty maintaining my focus on projects that take more than a few months to complete.***
   - ☐ Very much like me
   - ☐ Mostly like me
   - ☐ Somewhat like me
   - ☐ Not much like me
   - ☐ Not like me at all

7. **I finish whatever I begin.**
   - ☐ Very much like me
   - ☐ Mostly like me
   - ☐ Somewhat like me
   - ☐ Not much like me
   - ☐ Not like me at all

8. **I am diligent.**
- ☐ Very much like me
- ☐ Mostly like me
- ☐ Somewhat like me
- ☐ Not much like me
- ☐ Not like me at all

Scoring

For questions 2, 4, 7, and 8 assign the following points:

5 = Very much like me

4 = Mostly like me

3 = Somewhat like me

2 = Not much like me

1 = Not like me at all

* For questions 1, 3, 5, and 6 assign the following points:

1 = Very much like me

2 = Mostly like me

3 = Somewhat like me

4 = Not much like me

5 = Not like me at all

Add up all the points and divide by 8. The maximum score on this scale is 5 (extremely gritty), and the lowest score on this scale is 1 (not at all gritty).

Adapted from Duckworth and Quinn, 2009; (Duckworth, et al., 2007.)

Slips, Setbacks, and Relapse

I would be remiss if I did not address the research on slips, setbacks, and relapse as it relates to health behavior change. Unfortunately, relapse back to earlier stages of behavior change is the rule, rather than the exception. Research has shown that only 20 percent of the population actually conquers a long-term problem behavior and reaches *maintenance* of their new, positive behavior on the first attempt (Prochaska, et al., 2002). For example, the average smoker attempts to quit seven times before he or she is successful. This typically occurs because people jump into *action*, without the knowledge of the Stages of Change (Chapter 1) Processes of Change (Chapter 2), or don't leverage the other appropriate strategies, techniques, and tools described throughout this book. Some may not seek needed professional help for additional support for more deeply rooted issues such as strong, negative Core Beliefs (Chapter 5). One does not need to relapse from *action* or *maintenance* all the way down the change continuum to *precontemplation*. Remember: As noted in Chapter 1, "Change is a process" and "Change means *progress* (Prochaska, 2008). If we relapse from *action* to *contemplation* after having begun our journey at *precontemplation*, we have still made progress toward behavior change.

Examples of slips include picking up a cigarette and having an alcoholic drink ("falling off the wagon") after quitting. Slips are typically caused by overwhelming stress or inadequate coping skills (Prochaska, et al., 2002). If we do have a slip, it is important that we "get back on the horse" as quickly as possible. Eva-Molly Petitto Dunbar is a graduate student working on her doctoral dissertation research, under the direction of Dr. James Prochaska at the University of Rhode Island's Cancer Research Prevention Center (home of the Transtheoretical Model). Eva-Molly has extensive experience working with women with eating disorders, including the creation of the Eating Concerns Mentors Program, which she founded for University of New Hampshire college undergraduates (Dunbar, 2014), and where she observed students significantly struggling through the challenges of those pernicious "slips." She notes that a recommended strategy for women with eating disorders, such as binge eating, who slip on a meal and "binge," is to bounce back on the *very next* meal or snack. And there's a bright side to slipping! A slip may allow us to see what is going wrong and indicates that something is difficult, thus providing an opportunity to learn from the slip and to be more successful in the future. Many times after a slip, people will often say that they will resume eating healthfully, not smoking, not drinking, etc., on the Monday (or a later date) after a slip during the weekend or holiday. Here, setting a start date for *action* is great. However, if you are already in *action* and have a slip, the faster you can resume your healthy behavior, and the better chance you can avoid a more serious relapse back to a much earlier Stage of Change.

Thrive! The Ultimate End Zone

Positive psychology is based on the theory of well-being (Chapter 9). Its goal is to increase the degree to which one *flourishes or thrives* in his or her life, and the lives of others (Seligman, 2011; Cantril, 1965; Evers, et al., 2012). To thrive, one must possess the core elements of well-being (Chapter 9). Along with the core elements of well-being, positive self-esteem, optimism, resilience, vitality, and self-determination are very important traits of an individual who thrives or flourishes (Seligman, 2011).

Journal Activity

Ask yourself if the following statements describe you:

- In general, I feel very positive about myself (self-esteem).

- I'm always optimistic about my future (optimism).

- When things go wrong in my life, it doesn't take me long to bounce back (resilience).

- I feel physically and mentally strong, healthy, passionate, energetic, and zestful for life (vitality).

- I have a high degree of intrinsic motivation or am internally, not externally, motivated (self-determination).

Are you Thriving? Complete the Cantril Self-Anchoring Striving Scale

The Cantril Self-Anchoring Striving Scale was developed by a pioneering social researcher, Dr. Hadley Cantril, in 1965. It is a simple scale, however a highly effective and proven way to determine if you are thriving, struggling, or suffering (Evers, et al., 2012). As with life, your results may be variable, on any given day, so it is a good idea to re-assess on a regular basis to ensure you strive to or continue to thrive! To utilize the scale, imagine a ladder, with rungs numbered from 0 to 10. Zero is the bottom rung of the ladder, and 10 is the top rung. The top rung represents your best possible life; the bottom rung represents your worst possible life.

Ask yourself the following two questions:

1. On which rung of the ladder do I personally feel I am standing on at this given moment in time (present time)?
2. On which rung of the ladder do I personally feel I will stand in five years from now (in the future)?

Thriving

One is thriving if he or she rates his or her present position on rung 7 or higher on the ladder. Someone who rates his or her present position on rung 8 or higher has positive views of the present and future. Researchers have found that individuals who are thriving report significantly less health issues, more positive emotions and happiness, and more enjoyment and interest in life.

Struggling

For those who are struggling now or expect to be in the future, their well-being is at moderate risk and they rate their present life in the middle of the ladder, at rung 5 or 6. Well-being is inconsistent for those who are struggling. The respondents to the research performed on this scale report moderate views of their present life, or moderate or negative views of their future. They report more stress, illness, and concern about finances than thriving individuals. They also typically use double the amount of sick days than their thriving colleagues at work, and they are more likely to engage in unhealthy behaviors such as smoking or poor eating habits.

Suffering

One is suffering if he or she rates his or her life at rung 4 or below on the ladder. The well-being of someone who is suffering is at high risk. He or she has negative views about current life circumstances as well as the future, and may have less access to healthcare and basic necessities, such as food and shelter. Suffering individuals have more than double the burden of disease as compared to thriving respondents.

Individuals who are thriving are those with true grit and can be unstoppable. So can you! Remember: You got grit!

How do you learn how to or continue to thrive on the top rungs on the ladder? Apply the behavior change theories, and utilize the assessments, strategies, techniques, tools, and tips in this book!

The Seven Insider Secrets for Permanent Change

Continuously leverage the Seven Insider Secrets presented in this book on a daily basis. By doing so, you are less likely to have a slip or more likely to swiftly recover and prevent total relapse if you do.

1. **Insider Secret #1:** Am I ready to change? Assess and reassess your Stage of Change on a regular basis to increase your awareness and ensure you are leveraging the most effective Processes of Change.

2. **Insider Secret #2:** How do I start? Leverage the Processes of Change appropriate for your current Stage of Change.

3. **Insider Secret #3:** Return to Recess. Complete your activity history and commitment contract, Return to Recess daily, and have some fun!

4. **Insider Secret #4:** Building Confidence through Mastery. Use the Four Sources of Self-efficacy to improve your confidence to achieve your behavior change goals.

5. **Insider Secret #5:** Change the way you think about it. Monitor and change your thoughts to change your mind, change your health!

6. **Insider Secret #6:** Make a New Life Plan. Develop your mission, vision, SMART goals, and personal behavior change plan. Self-manage and monitor your progress daily.

7. **Insider Secret #7:** Game On! Leverage the powerful strategies from sports psychology to keep you charged and ready for action!

In addition to the Seven Insider Secrets to behavior change, utilize the assessments, strategies, and techniques in Sustaining Change (Part II):

- Push through lifecycle events by applying the keys to sustaining change through challenging times.
- Practice the ways to well-being on a daily basis.
- Remember: You got grit!

Call to ACTION: Be a Wellness Rock Star!

In my book *Winning Health Promotion Strategies*, I describe an introduction that occurred following a presentation I made at a conference in Washington, D.C. A close colleague introduced me to someone in the audience from my home state of Rhode Island. The man quickly responded to my colleague, "I know Annie, the Rock Star of Wellness!" We all chuckled at this interesting response. As the former director of the governor's Wellness Initiative in Rhode Island, I had the opportunity to work with many representatives of the wellness and healthcare industries, along with businesses, in the smallest state in the union, as well as other states across the country. Although I met a lot of people and established a national network, I hardly considered myself a rock star!

Afterward, as a music lover, I realized there is much more to being a rock star than being recognizable and notoriety. Rock stars *inspire* people. They have the ability to motivate and, in some cases, move people toward change in their life, through their craft. When many of us listen to a musician or rock star, we experience vivid memories of some of the most challenging, and joyous lifecycle events of our lives. Through their lyrics and inspiring performances, rock stars connect with millions of people and inspire and influence many individuals to make significant, life altering changes. We can learn a great deal from rock stars as we strive to inspire and move ourselves and others toward positive change and engagement in healthy lifestyle behaviors. Throughout my 30-year career in the health and wellness industry, I have had the privilege and pleasure of working with and meeting many rock stars of wellness. Whether working in the health and wellness industry or not, rock stars inspire themselves *and* others toward change. So, this is a call to action. I challenge you to be a rock star of wellness! Inspire yourself to *change your mind, change your health,* and provide the social support and encouragement to inspire *others* to make healthy lifestyle changes. So, let's rock on!

(Adapted from *Winning Health Promotion Strategies.*)

Key Points

- Grit is defined as the combination of strong perseverance and a deep passion to achieve an objective or goal.
- Achievement = skill times (x) effort.
- "Got grit" is posed as a statement versus a question, as we *all* already have a degree of this powerful trait. Its power simply needs to be harnessed!
- Slips, setbacks, and relapse are the rule rather than the exception. Prepare for them to be the exception.
- Review the Seven Insider Secrets regularly to maintain your behavior change progress.
- Thrive: your ultimate end zone!

Action Items

- Complete the Grit Scale.
- Perform the Journal Activities.
- Continuously leverage the Seven Insider Secrets.
- Push through lifecycle events by applying the keys to sustaining change through challenging times.
- Practice the ways to well-being on a daily basis.
- Strengthen your Grit.
- Complete the Cantril Self-Anchoring Striving Scale.
- Answer the Call to Action: Be a Wellness Rock Star!

References

Algoe, S.B., and B.L. Fredrickson. "Emotional fitness and the movement of affective science from lab to field." *The American Psychologist* 66, no. 1 (2011): 35–42.

American Psychological Association. *The Road to Resilience.* (2004). *www.apa.org/helpcenter/road-resilience.aspx#.*

Aten, J., K. O'Grady, and E. Worthington, eds. *Psychology of Religion and Research Spirituality for Clinicians: Using Research in Your Practice.* New York: Routledge, Taylor and Francis Group, 2011.

Bachorowski, J.A. and M.J. Owren. "Not all laughs are alike: voiced but not unvoiced laughter readily elicits positive affect." *Psychological Science: A Journal of the American Psychological Society* 12, no. 3 (2001): 252–257.

Bandura, A. *Self-Efficacy: The Exercise of Control.* New York: Freeman, 1997.

Beck, J.S. *Cognitive Behavior Therapy: Basics and Beyond.* New York: Guilford Press, 2011.

Berrigan, D.K., R.P. Troiano, S.M. Krebs-Smith, and R.B. Barbash. "Patterns of health behavior in U.S. adults." *Preventive Medicine* 36, vol. 5 (2003): 615–623.

Bonanno, G.A. "Loss, trauma, and human resilience: have we underestimated the human capacity to thrive after extremely aversive events?" *The American Psychologist* 59, vol. 1 (2004): 20–28.

Buettner, D. *The Blue Zones: Lessons for Living Longer from the People Who've Lived the Longest.* Washington, D.C.: National Geographic Society, 2010.

Burton, D., and T. Raedeke. *Sport Psychology for Coaches.* Champaign, Ill.: Human Kinetics, 2008.

Cantril, H. *The Pattern of Human Concerns.* New Brunswick, N.J.: Rutgers University Press, 1965.

Centers for Disease Control and Prevention. "Current Cigarette Smoking Among Adults." *MMWR* 63, vol. 2 (2014): 29–34.

Chandler, S. *100 Ways to Motivate Yourself: Change Your Life Forever.* Pompton Plains, N.J.: Career Press, 2012.

Cohn, M.A., B.L. Fredrickson, S.L. Brown, J.A. Mikels, and A.M. Conway. "Happiness unpacked: positive emotions increase life satisfaction by building resilience." *Emotion* 9, no. 3 (2009): 361–368.

Cox, R.H. *Sport Psychology: Concepts and Applications.* New York: McGraw-Hill, 2012.

Cox, H.R., Y. Qiu, and Z. Liu. "Overview of sport psychology" in R.N. Singer, M. Murphey, and L.K. Tennant, eds. *Handbook of Research on Sport Psychology.* New York: Maxwell Macmillan International, 1993.

Diener, E. "Subjective well-being. The science of happiness and a proposal for a national index." *The American Psychologist* 55, no. 1 (2000): 34–43.

Diener, E., R.A. Emmons, R.J. Larsen, and S. Griffin. "The Satisfaction With Life Scale." *Journal of Personality Assessment* 49, no. 1 (1985): 71–75.

Dillon, K., B. Minchoff, and K.H. Baker. "Positive emotional states and enhancement of the immune system." *International Journal of Psychiatry in Medicine* 15 (1985–1986): 13–18.

Duckworth, A.L, and P.D. Quinn. "Development and validation of the Short Grit Scale (Grit- S)." *Journal of Personality Assessment* 91 (2009): 166–174.

Duckworth, A.L., C. Peterson, M.D. Matthews, and D.R. Kelly. "Grit: perseverance and passion for long-term goals." *Journal of Personality and Social Psychology* 92, no. 6 (2007): 1087–1101.

Dunbar, E-M.P. *Evaluating the impact of a college-based Eating Concerns Mentors (ECM) program on improvements to body image: Implications for the prevention of eating disorders.* Manuscript submitted for publication. (2014).

Evers, K.E., J.O. Prochaska, P.H. Castle, J.L. Johnson, J.M. Prochaska, P.L. Harrison, and E.J. Pope. "Development of an individual well-being scores assessment." *Psychology of Well-Being: Theory, Research and Practice* 2 vol. 2 (2012): doi:10.1186/2211-1522-2-2.

Fleig, L., S. Lippke, S. Pomp, and R. Schwarzer. "Exercise maintenance after rehabilitation: How experience can make a difference." *Psychology of Sport and Exercise* 12 (2011): 293–299.

Foulds, H.J., S.S.D. Bredin, S. Charlesworth, S.A.C. Ivey, and D.E.R. Warburton. "Exercise volume and intensity: a dose-response relationship with health benefits." *European Journal of Applied Physiology.* (2014).

Fredrickson, B.L., M.M. Tugade, C.E. Waugh, and G.R. Larkin. "What good are positive emotions in crisis? A prospective study of resilience and emotion following the terrorist attacks on the United States on September 11th, 2001." *Journal of Personality and Social Psychology* 84 (2003): 365–376.

Gucciardi, D.F., S. Gordon, and J.A. Dimmock. "Advancing mental toughness research and theory using personal construct psychology." *International Review of Sport and Exercise Psychology* 2 (2009): 54–72.

Holmes, T.H. and R.H. Rahe. "The social readjustment rating scale." *Journal of Psychosomatic Research* 11 (1967): 213–218.

Hobbis, I.C.A. and S. Sutton. "Are techniques used in cognitive behaviour therapy applicable to behaviour change interventions based on the theory of planned behaviour? *Journal of Health Psychology* 10, vol. 1 (2005). 7–18, 37–43.

Hope, D.A., J.A. Burns, S.A. Hayes, J.D. Herbert, and M.D. Warner. "Automatic Thoughts and Cognitive Restructuring in Cognitive Behavioral Group Therapy for Social Anxiety Disorder." *Cognitive Therapy and Research.* (2010).

Hofmann, W., M. Friese, and F. Strack. "Impulse and self-control from a dual-systems perspective." *Perspectives on Psychological Science.* (2009).

Jayawickreme, E., M.J.C. Forgeard, and M.E.P. Seligman. "The engine of well-being." *American Psychological Association* 16 (2012): 327–342.

Johnson, S.S., A.L. Paiva, L. Mauriello, J.O. Prochaska, C. Redding, and W.F. Velicer. "Coaction in Multiple Behavior Change Interventions: Consistency Across Multiple Studies on Weight Management and Obesity Prevention." *Health Psychology: Official Journal of the Division of Health Psychology, American Psychological Association.* (2013).

Karageorghis, C.I., and D.L. Priest. "Music in the exercise domain: a review and synthesis (Part II)." *International Review of Sport and Exercise Psychology.* (2012).

Ludovici-Connolly, A.M. *Winning Health Promotion Strategies.* Champaign, Ill.: Human Kinetics, 2010.

Masuda, A., S.C. Hayes, C.F. Sackett, and M.P. Twohig. "Cognitive defusion and self-relevant negative thoughts: Examining the impact of a ninety year old technique." *Behaviour Research and Therapy* 42, vol. 4 (2004): 477–485.

Miller, W.R., and R.K. Hester. "Treating the problem drinker: Modern approaches" in *The Addictive Behavior: Treatment of Alcoholism, Drug Abuse, Smoking and Obesity*, W.R. Miller, ed., Oxford: Pergamon Press, 1980.

Norcross, J.C., M.S. Mrykalo, and M.D. Blagys. "Auld lang syne: success predictors, change processes, and self-reported outcomes of New Year's resolvers and nonresolvers." *Journal of Clinical Psychology* 58, vol. 4 (2002): 397–405.

Olson, R., S. Schmidt, C. Winkler, and B. Wipfli. "The effects of target behavior choice and self-management skills training on compliance with behavioral self-monitoring." *American Journal of Health Promotion* 25 vol. 5 (2011): 319–324.

O'Reilly, N. "Wellbeing: The five essential elements." *The Journal of Positive Psychology* 8 no. 2 (2013): 174–176.

Pajares, F., and T.C. Urdan. *Self-Efficacy Beliefs of Adolescents.* Greenwich, Conn.: Information Age Publishing, 2006.

Prochaska, J.O. "Multiple health behavior research represents the future of preventive medicine." *Preventive Medicine* 46 (2008): 583–602.

Prochaska, J.O., J.C. Norcross, and C.C. DiClemente. *Changing for Good.* New York: Quill, 2002.

Prochaska, J.O., C.A. Redding, and K. Evers. "The Transtheoretical Model and Stages of Change" in K. Glanz, B.K. Rimer, and F.M. Lewis, eds. *Health Behavior and Health Education: Theory, Research, and Practice.* San Francisco, Calif.: Jossey-Bass, Inc., 2002.

Prochaska, J.O., and W.F. Velicer. "The transtheoretical model of health behavior change." *American Journal of Health Promotion* 12, vol. 1 (1997): 38–48.

Sallis, J.F., and M.F. Hovell. "Determinants of exercise behavior." *Exercise and Sport Sciences Reviews* 18 (1990): 307–330.

Sallis, J.F., M.F. Hovell, and C.R. Hofstetter. "Predictors of adoption and maintenance of vigorous physical activity in men and women." *Preventive Medicine* 21 (1992): 237–251.

Seligman, M.E.P. *Flourish: A Visionary New Understanding of Happiness and Well-Being.* New York: Free Press, 2011.

Seligman, M.E., M. Csikszentmihalyi. "Positive psychology. An introduction." *The American Psychologist* 55, vol. 1 (2000): 5–14.

Sun, X., J.O. Prochaska, W.F. Velicer, and R.G. Laforge. "Transtheoretical principles and processes for quitting smoking: A 24-month comparison of a representative sample of quitters, relapsers, and non-quitters." *Addictive Behaviors* 32, no. 12 (2007): 2707–2726.

Warner, L.M., B. Schüz, K. Knittle, J.P. Ziegelmann, and S. Wurm. "Sources of perceived self-efficacy as predictors of physical activity in older adults." *Applied Psychology: Health and Well-Being* 3 (2011): 172–192.

Weinberg, R.S., and D. Gould. *Foundations of Sport and Exercise Psychology.* Champaign, Ill.: Human Kinetics, 2011.

Williams, J.M., and V. Krane. "Psychological characteristics of peak performance" in J. Williams, ed., *Applied Sport Psychology: Personal Growth to Peak Performance.* Mountain View, Calif.: Mayfield Publishing Company, 1998.

Index

About the Author

Anne Marie Ludovici (Annie) is a noted author, speaker, well-being activist, and leading authority in affective personal lifestyle enrichment. Annie helps people change—from the inside out, and her best-selling book, *Winning Health Promotions Strategies,* is considered the blueprint for fostering healthy communities everywhere. With a masters in kinesiology and a major in Psychology and social aspects of behavior change, Annie has been at the forefront 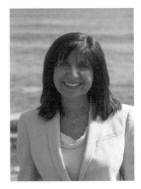 of numerous pioneering state and national wellness initiatives. Working with today's leading minds in health and wellness, along with human behavior, Annie blends academic theory with more than 30 years of health and wellness experience to empower meaningful, personal, life-enriching changes that last. Her unique expertise and proven methodology have helped a wide range of clients—from Fortune 100 clients to small businesses, heathcare providers, and state and local governments—make a change for the healthier. Annie lives in Wakefield, Rhode Island.